Praise for *Ayurveda Beginner's Guide* by Susan Weis-Bohlen

"Reading *Ayurveda Beginner's Guide* feels like a friend taking your hand and warmly guiding you to feeling a lot better. It's a wonderful and helpful book."
—**SHARON SALZBERG**, *New York Times*-bestselling author of *Real Happiness* and *Real Love*

"*Ayurveda Beginner's Guide* will take you on an effortless journey into the world of Ayurveda that promises to change your life, as it has mine!"
—**DR. JOHN DOUILLARD, DC, CAP**, Founder of LifeSpa.com and bestselling author of *Eat Wheat* and *The 3-Season Diet*

"Susan Weis-Bohlen has provided a practical and user-friendly introduction and guide to Ayurveda for the health-conscious seekers of balanced living."
—**HILARY GIRAVALTIS**, executive director of the National Ayurvedic Medical Association and founder of the Kripalu School of Ayurveda

"Susan Weis-Bohlen has translated the ancient healing system of Ayurveda into real-world, practical applications. Each page of this beautiful book lovingly guides us with profound yet easy-to-apply steps that bring our bodies back to a state of wholeness, our minds back into the present moment, and our Souls to a more peaceful vibration. *Ayurveda Beginner's Guide* is a powerful, comprehensive blueprint for living a healthy, balanced, and abundant life, and I am grateful to her for sharing this timeless wisdom in such an accessible format."
—**DAVIDJI**, Author of *Secrets of Meditation* (Nautilus Book Award winner)

"Susan Weis-Bohlen has a deep understanding of what is one of the world's oldest systems of medicine. She also has a unique talent for translating her knowledge of Ayurveda so that both health professionals and lay readers can gain more insight and understanding."
—**BRIAN BERMAN, MD**, director of the University of Maryland School of Medicine Center for Integrative Medicine, founder and president of the Institute for Integrative Health

"*Ayurveda Beginner's Guide* introduces readers to concepts and practices that can be added to one's daily living right away. Susan Weis-Bohlen also shares deeper aspects of this powerful healing path that she has learned and practiced over the years. This book is a guide to how ancient Eastern practices can have a healing impact in the West today."
—**DR. RAMKUMAR KUTTY**, co-founder of Vaidyagrama Ayurvedic Healing Village (Vaidyagrama.com) and Punarnava Trust, India (Punarnava.org)

"*Ayurveda Beginner's Guide* by Susan Weis-Bohlen is a gem. For those who are looking to learn more about the ancient, healing powers of Ayurveda, look no further than this wonderful resource."

—**REBECCA KATZ, MS**, author of *The Cancer-Fighting Kitchen*

"If you're looking for a new way to pursue health and wisdom, this book is your answer. Beautiful and vibrant, *Ayurveda Beginner's Guide* welcomes you to an ancient path for healing. Filled with practical, doable advice for everyday living, it's accessible, clear, engaging, and so encouraging. Your travel guide for the journey, Susan Weis-Bohlen, lives this path and walks her talk. She, too, was a beginner once and takes you on this journey with lively compassion and practical humor. Go for it!"

—**AMADEA MORNINGSTAR**, author of *Easy Healing Drinks from the Wisdom of Ayurveda* (AmadeaMorningstar.net)

"As a physician who practices Ayurveda, I am always asked by patients for resources that will help them delve into this beautiful and ancient science. I am truly grateful that Susan Weis-Bohlen has taken her many years of wisdom and compiled it into an easy-to-use handbook. *Ayurveda Beginner's Guide* includes an overview of dosha types, lifestyle practices, dietary guidelines, recipes, yoga poses, and other balancing Ayurvedic treatments. The writing is clear and concise, and I know this book will help many readers use this ancient medicine to achieve a more optimal way of living."

—**TRUPTI GOKANI, MD**, award-winning, board-certified neurologist (TruptiGokanimd.com)

"In *Ayurveda Beginner's Guide*, Susan Weis-Bohlen skillfully translates the empowering teachings of this ancient system of wellness for a modern-day audience. Her enthusiasm for and knowledge of the artistry of Ayurveda shines forth on every page. User-friendly and approachable, this guide is a must-have for anyone interested in Ayurveda."

—**FELICIA TOMASKO, RN**, editor-in-chief of *LA Yoga Ayurveda and Health* magazine, former member of the National Ayurvedic Medical Association board of directors, and former president of California Association of Ayurvedic Medicine

"Clearly and concisely, Susan Weis-Bohlen offers a comprehensive introduction to Ayurveda, deftly mixing her own experience following Ayurvedic principles with explanations of its approach, long history, and range of benefits. The tone is serious, helpful and sometimes funny (as when the digestive tract tries to figure out what to do with ingested Cheez Doodles). This detailed book—full of recipes, information about yoga, meditation, medicine, and more—makes it easy for anyone to learn about Ayurveda."

—**JOHN MUTTER**, editor-in-chief and co-founder of *Shelf Awareness*

AYURVEDA BEGINNER'S GUIDE

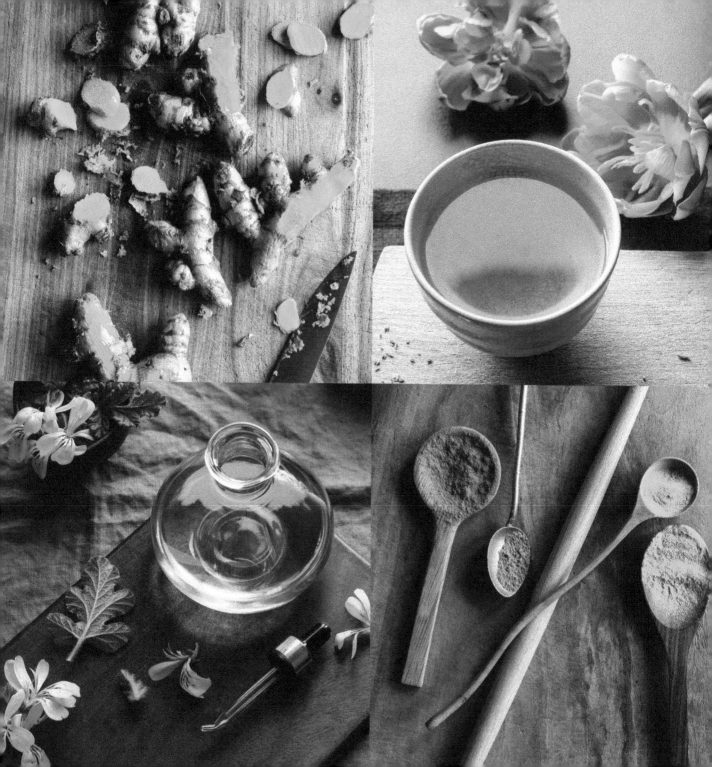

AYURVEDA
BEGINNER'S GUIDE

Essential Ayurvedic Principles & Practices
to Balance & Heal Naturally

Susan Weis-Bohlen

ROCKRIDGE
PRESS

For general information on our other products and services, please contact our Customer Care Department within the United States at (866) 744-2665, or outside the United States at (510) 253-0500.

Paperback ISBN: 978-1-939754-17-2
eBook ISBN: 978-1-939754-19-6

Manufactured in the United States of America

Photography © Nadine Greeff, 2018; Hélène Dujardin, cover; Alita Ong/Stocksy, cover.

10 9 8 7 6 5 4 3

To my partner in Ayurveda,
life, and love, my heart—Larry

CONTENTS

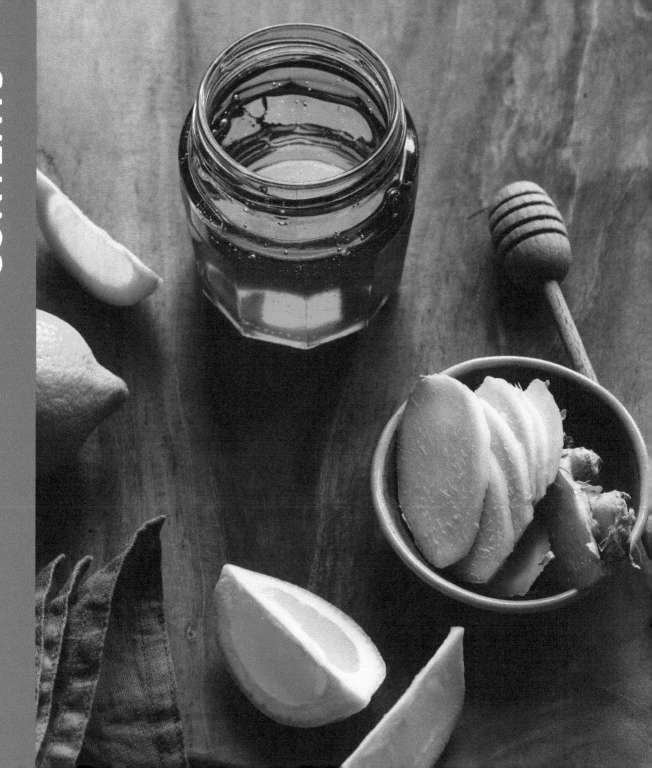

INTRODUCTION

In 2004, I opened a metaphysical bookstore in my hometown of Baltimore, Maryland. Although business was sailing along, I felt unsatisfied in a few core areas of my life, including my health and relationships. I began to think about a way forward that would be more fulfilling and sustainable. The answer came to me in 2007 in the form of Ayurveda.

Before I embraced Ayurveda, my weight had always been an issue for me; I began dieting when I was only 14 years old. I also struggled with bulimia on and off for years, losing and gaining weight so often that I finally decided not to think about it anymore. I did not lead an unhappy life, though. I traveled the world, lived overseas for a while, and had amazing adventures. Although I'd reached nearly 220 pounds, my weight didn't stand in my way, but it didn't help me either.

By the time I opened my store, I felt stuffed, not only with food, but also with thoughts, plans, ideas, and desires. Even though I had been eating a vegetarian diet, meditating regularly, and attending yoga class for years, I still felt that I was holding myself back from my full potential. Then in August 2007, I led a small group of travelers to England on a sacred site tour. During the tour, as I stood in a crop circle, a knowing came over me that I had to be open to creating room in my life for something new, in whatever way it came to me. Later in the trip, I buried two small pieces of rose quartz under a rock at the standing stones in Avebury. Mentally noting where they were, I vowed to retrieve them as a healthier woman whose body and mind truly reflected how I felt, and who enjoyed a solid relationship with the man I would be spending the rest of my life with.

Back home in Baltimore, I began to listen deep within myself for a message on how to feel better, and I found myself yearning for a cleanse. I wanted to rid myself of anything that stood in the way of my health and well-being. As I began to research cleansing practices, I came across the Ayurvedic term *panchakarma*, which translates to "five actions." As I read, I learned that panchakarma is a series of treatments that cleanses the body and rebuilds the tissues.

This ancient Indian practice resonated with me so deeply that I booked a flight to San Diego, California, to visit the Chopra Center for a week of panchakarma and classes on Ayurveda, the traditional system of Indian medicine. During my stay at the Chopra Center, toxins began to loosen up and flow out of me, physically and emotionally, creating space for whatever was to come next. I returned home feeling that a deeply profound shift had occurred within me, and I planned to embrace it.

I had a small Ayurvedic section in my bookstore, including some great Ayurvedic cookbooks. (In Ayurveda, food is medicine, so cooking nutritious food is the backbone of the practice.) I took home a collection of books and immersed myself in their pages. With this knowledge behind me, I went to an Indian market and bought the starter items I needed for a kitchen that would help me create healing foods to balance my mind and body. When I returned, I made the first of many *kitcharis*, vegetarian stew made with mung beans and rice, considered one of the most healing Ayurvedic foods. I also bought oils and herbal supplements to continue the practices I had learned.

As I began to approach the world through the Ayurvedic principles you will learn about in this book, everything began to make more sense to me, and the results I experienced were rapid and encouraging. In fewer than three months, I dropped nearly 30 pounds, and my cholesterol fell an astonishing 80 points. (In all, I have lost over 60 pounds.) Other areas of my life that hadn't been serving me started changing as well. For instance, I sought out corners of my house where clutter had accumulated over the years and threw away the unwanted items. I created more breathing space and felt the *prana*, or life force, flowing through me and around me.

As my life shifted in large and small ways, I wanted to share these transformative Ayurvedic principles with others, so I signed up for the Chopra Center's Teacher Certification program. This course supplied me with an organized path of study. I also began to study Ayurvedic cooking with seminal Ayurvedic cookbook author Amadea Morningstar. Through Amadea's wisdom, I learned cooking techniques and beautiful practices to use while cooking. Over the past decade, I have also worked and studied with Dr. Vasant Lad of the Ayurvedic Institute in New Mexico and India.

In 2014, I closed my shop to focus on my new path. I now have a full-time practice as an Ayurvedic consultant, cooking teacher, meditation teacher, and leader of sacred site tours. And, of course, three years after I buried those stones at Avebury, England, I did return as a new woman with my amazing fiancé by my side. We couldn't locate the pieces of rose quartz I'd buried, but I had kept the promise I made!

Like I once did with the many books in my shop, you are reading this book because you are interested in learning about how Ayurveda can help you feel better. You may have come to the end of your rope with the conventional health-care system and have turned here for ideas, remedies, insights, and ancient wisdom you can start using today. This book explores the various reasons why this system may be the best answer for whatever ails you— physically, mentally, and emotionally. Small changes can have profound effects, so begin your path by trying out some of the recipes and practices for a few weeks. Everything you need to know to get started is within.

PART ONE

An Ancient System of Healing

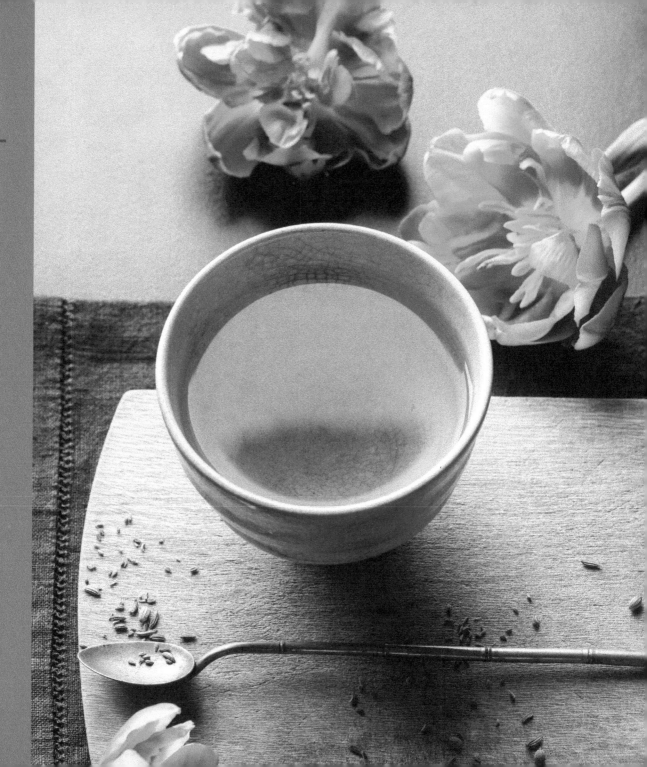

CHAPTER 1

An Overview of Ayurveda

While it just isn't possible to boil down 5,000 years of teachings into a single book, the good news is that you don't need to know everything to start welcoming Ayurveda into your life and benefiting from its practices. In this chapter, you will be introduced to some of the key concepts and you will assess your unique mind-body type within the Ayurvedic system of health and healing. Once you know your type, the rest will fall into place—and you won't have to remember the esoteric terms, because even the basic concepts are profound.

WHAT IS AYURVEDA?

Often viewed as the first system of medicine ever established, Ayurveda is a 5,000-year-old Indian system of care that holistically addresses the mind, body, and spirit. It emphasizes eating right to bring yourself back into balance, exercising, breathing fully, reducing stress, sleeping well, and other basic concepts to keep your body whole, balanced, and healthy.

In Ayurveda, food is medicine. When a person eats in a manner that is best for their unique needs, they can improve their health, live longer, and protect themselves from disease. Other Ayurvedic practices further support a strong mind-body constitution. While all of the Ayurvedic practices help you maintain good health, if you do get sick, the thought is that you can heal faster because your body is in better balance.

Knowledge of Ayurveda comes from the Vedas, which originated in India, and are some of the oldest written texts in the world. This system of medicine was taught to students who visited the great teachers of India (the *rishis*) to learn from them. The science of life, which Ayurveda is often called, was originally an oral tradition transmitted through concepts and poetic phrases (*sutras*, literally meaning "thread") that were used to pass knowledge from one generation to the next. Even today, an Ayurvedic doctor may sing a sutra to explain a treatment or impart wisdom.

Many forms of medicine have roots in Ayurveda. For instance, herbal medicine, energy medicine, traditional Chinese medicine (TCM), polarity therapy, marma therapy, acupuncture, acupressure, and even Reiki and healing touch are either used in Ayurveda or share something in common with this system. That is one reason Ayurveda is so accepting of integrative medicine. It recognizes that there is wisdom to be found in many traditions.

Who Can Benefit from Ayurveda?

Ayurveda is a versatile system of health care because it can be tailored to suit any person's unique needs. Following an Ayurvedic lifestyle can help people stay healthy, recover faster from illness, and hopefully set the stage for a long life. It can also complement traditional medicine for those who are already unwell or on medications and become an integrative part of their health-care support system.

If Ayurveda can do so much for so many people, and has a history of use for over 5,000 years, why isn't it a more common approach to health and wellness? Truth is, people tend to lean toward more modern concepts of health and healing, thinking that if it's newer, it must be superior. This isn't always true. After reading this book and trying out these practices, you may conclude that this ancient understanding of mind-body balance might even be more advanced than today's established health-care system.

Ayurveda and Religion

Many people think of Ayurveda and yoga as Hindu practices, and worry that it will conflict with their religious traditions. I came to Ayurveda as a Jewish woman who had been practicing Buddhist meditation for years. I had no idea that Ayurveda had any relationship to Hinduism. I certainly didn't need to be Hindu to incorporate Ayurvedic practices into my life and benefit from them. However, I do find the Hindu religion fascinating, beautiful, and filled with stories and texts like the *Bhagavad Gita* and the *Upanishads* that are as relevant today as they were thousands of years ago.

You can have a powerful Ayurvedic practice without immersing yourself in Hinduism or learning Sanskrit (the classical language of India) or having statues of Hindu gods and goddesses like Ganesh (the remover of obstacles) around your house. Someday, you may want to know more about Ayurveda, its sister sciences, and ancient texts, but first take your time with this book. You may discover you benefit enough from just the practices found in this book.

Ayurveda's Story of Creation

There is an ancient story of how Ayurveda was introduced to the world: When the gods (*devas*) and demons (*asuras*) created the world, they each wanted to achieve immortality. By pulling on a rope attached to a pole that was anchored to a giant tortoise, they churned a bowl containing an ocean of milk. The churning produced the nectar of the gods, called *Amrita* or *Soma*—immortality, longevity, perfect health. From this churning arose the "divine physician" named Dhanvantari (avatar of the Hindu Lord Vishnu), holding a bowl of the elixir, Soma. Now known as the God of Ayurveda, Dhanvantari holds the bowl for all those who practice Ayurveda to drink from.

THE UNIVERSE OF AYURVEDA

An underlying principle of Ayurveda is that we are both energy and matter combined. Each of us, as well as our environment, is made up of the five great elements (*Maha Bhutas*): (1) Space, (2) Air, (3) Fire, (4) Water, and (5) Earth. These are the building blocks of our world. They create our foundation and structure (earth); movement and circulation (air and space); transformation, light, and metabolism (fire); and cohesiveness, digestive juices, and secretions (water).

The five great elements are found in varying amounts in every person and the environment. Some people and places will have more of one element than another. Think of the desert as having more fire (heat) and air (dryness), the beach as having more water, and the mountains as having more earth. Likewise, some of us are more "earthy," some us are more "spacey," and others are more "intense" or "hot." Our unique combination of the five elements makes up our predominant body composition, or *dosha*, of which there are three types: Vata, Pitta, and Kapha. (See Your Unique Body Composition [Your Dosha] on page 7.) Here are the qualities associated with each of the five great elements:

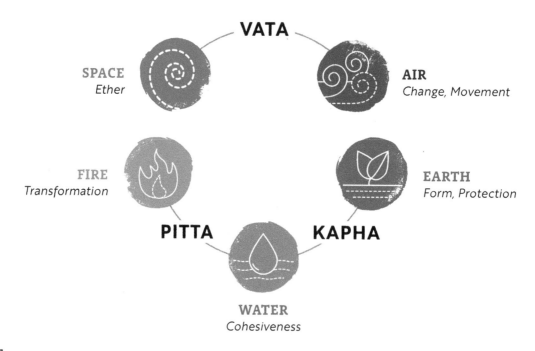

VATA

SPACE
Ether

AIR
Change, Movement

FIRE
Transformation

EARTH
Form, Protection

PITTA

KAPHA

WATER
Cohesiveness

Your Unique Body Composition (Your Dosha)

Your unique mind-body constitution, or dosha, comprises the five great elements. The way these elements present themselves at birth depends upon many things, including where you were conceived and born, how the planets were aligned at your birth, the state of mind of your parents when you were conceived, the food they ate prior to conceiving you, and even your past lives.

The primary dosha you are born with is known as your *prakruti*. As we grow, we typically enter into a state of imbalance, or *vikruti*, due to the influences of our environment, the food we eat, the emotional state of our home, and so on. By adopting the practices of Ayurveda, you can move yourself slowly but surely back toward your natural way of being, your prakruti.

The three doshas are Vata, Pitta, and Kapha. Although one dosha is usually dominant, each of us is made up of all three. In the next section, you will find a simple quiz that can help you identify your dosha, and then you can review the chart on page 10, which includes a brief rundown of the characteristics of each dosha, including signs of balance and imbalance.

When the doshas are disturbed by a person's lifestyle choices and/or environmental conditions, signs of imbalance manifest in both the mind and body. An imbalance can result in a disease or a general feeling of being unwell. The idea isn't to bring all three doshas into equal balance within you. The goal is to be the best unique makeup of yourself that you can be. You can do that by keeping your doshic balance in check through the Ayurvedic practices you will learn in part 2.

DOSHA QUIZ

To help determine your dosha, choose one of the three choices that best describes you. If you are tossed between two choices, ask someone for their opinion of how they might describe that particular quality.

BODY SIZE
A. I have a thin build.
B. I have a medium build.
C. I have a large build.

WEIGHT
A. I tend to have a low body weight. It's difficult to keep weight on.
B. My weight is normal. I've maintained my general weight for the last 10 years.
C. I am on the heavy side. It's difficult for me to lose weight.

HAIR
A. My hair is thin and dry, frizzy, brittle.
B. My hair is fine and prone to early graying.
C. My hair is thick and full and a little oily.

SKIN
A. My skin is thin; I can see my veins. I tend to have dry skin and wrinkles.
B. My skin is warm. My cheeks are red and warm to the touch. I am prone to skin problems.
C. My skin is thick; I cannot see my veins. It is cold or cool to the touch, and smooth with few wrinkles.

EYES
A. I have small eyes; they tend to dart around. I don't hold a steady gaze.
B. I have an intense and penetrating gaze. I tend to look directly at people.
C. My eyes are large and pleasant. I tend to gaze warmly at people.

TONGUE/MOUTH
A. My tongue is thin and can have a dark coating. I tend to have a dry mouth; my lips dry out and crack.
B. My tongue is rosy, medium thick, and pointy and can have a yellowish coating. I have a warm, moist mouth; my lips are thin and reddish, and tend to get inflamed.
C. My tongue is thick and rounded and can have a white coating. My lips are smooth, moist, and thick.

JOINTS

A. My joints creak and crack. I am bony and not very flexible.

B. I am flexible and have loose joints.

C. My joints are well lubricated and thickly padded.

NAILS

A. My nails crack and can split easily. They are dry and thin. The nail bed is whitish.

B. My nails are flexible. They tend to grow long. The nail bed is reddish.

C. My nails are strong, thick, and shiny with a large cuticle.

BODY TEMPERATURE

A. I tend to feel cold even on hot days.

B. I feel hot. I wear shorts and T-shirts, even in cold weather.

C. I feel comfortable in most climates, but I most dislike cold, damp days.

WHEN STRESSED

A. I have butterflies in my tummy. I am anxious and worried. I forget to eat. I blame myself when things go wrong.

B. I get agitated and frustrated. I feel impatient with myself and others. I blame others when things go wrong.

C. I withdraw. I overeat. I blame myself or others when things go wrong, but I convince others that nothing is wrong.

USUAL MOOD

A. I am spontaneous, enthusiastic, and lively. I am fine with change.

B. I am intense and purposeful. I like to convince people. I get easily frustrated with others. I like things to go my way.

C. I am easygoing, good-natured, and calm. I like routine. I tend to nurture others, sometimes at the risk of not caring for myself.

SLEEP PATTERNS/DREAMS

A. I awaken easily, and it is hard to get back to sleep. I have flying dreams. Some of my dreams are filled with anxiety and worry.

B. I sleep for short periods of time and feel rested. I dream of challenges, competition, heat, and fire.

C. I sleep deeply, sometimes 10 hours or more, and it is difficult to wake up. My dreams are slow, easygoing, romantic, and caring.

Results ➤

Mostly A's indicate **Vata**.

Mostly B's indicate **Pitta**.

Mostly C's indicate **Kapha**.

Even the difference of one number in your total reveals your dosha. For instance, if you choose 7 A's and 5 B's, you are Vata. If you choose an equal amount of two doshas, you may be bi-doshic, so pay particular attention to the seasonal suggestions in chapter 8. An equal number of A's, B's, and C's is tri-doshic; only a small percentage fit into this category. If you do, you will need to pay particular attention to the changes in season to keep your doshas in balance. To be sure that you are bi- or tri-doshic, ask someone to answer the questions in the quiz for you, and total those answers for a double-check.

OVERVIEW OF DOSHA CHARACTERISTICS

VATA (MOVEMENT)	PITTA (TRANSFORMATION)	KAPHA (PROTECTION)
DESCRIPTION		
Space and Air create transportation, movement, moves like the wind	Fire and Water create transformation, metabolism, heat up the body and mind	Earth and Water create protection, structure, stability
SEASON		
Fall and early winter	Summer	Late winter and spring
GENERAL CHARACTERISTICS		
Airy, cold, dry, fast, irregular, light, mobile, rough, spacey, unpredictable	Acidic, hot, intense, light, penetrating, sharp, sour	Cold, oily, slow, sluggish, smooth, solid, stable, steady, moist

PHYSICAL ATTRIBUTES

Thin; Light frame; Delicate digestion; Cold hands and feet; Irregular sleep patterns; Dry skin and hair; Moves and talks quickly; Resists routine; Loves new experiences (Think Calista Flockhart, Uma Thurman, Fred Astaire)

Medium build; Strong digestion; Warm body temp; Sleeps soundly for short periods (and loves to tell you this!); Sharp intellect; Learns very quickly; Direct in speech and action; Intense; Sharp; Stays close to routine; Courageous; Perfectionist and expects this in others (Think Lance Armstrong, Denzel Washington, Nicole Kidman)

Can be heavyset; Hearty stamina (rarely gets sick); Cold body temp; Deep, sound sleep; Smooth skin and thick hair; Solid; Stable; Smooth; Steady; Slow moving; Easygoing; Methodical; Sweet; Caring; Enjoys routine (Think Oprah, John Goodman, Rachael Ray)

SIGNS OF BALANCE

Can adapt quickly; Excitable and affectionate; Highly energetic; Incredibly creative; Loves to meet new people; Sees outside the box; Speaks up; Spontaneous

Courageous; Direct in speech and action; Friendly; Great leader; Intense; Likes routine; Quick to learn; Sharp intellect; Warm personality

Calm; Consistent; Content; Loyal; Steady; Strong; Supportive

SIGNS OF IMBALANCE

Often late; Anxiety, fear, and worry; Blames self and gets confused, anxious, and fearful when sad or depressed; Forgets to eat; Constipation; Difficulty finishing projects; Easily distracted; Extremely talkative; Gas, bloating; Insomnia; Overactive mind—constant chatter; Unfocused

Aggressive; Angry; Blames others and lashes out when sad or depressed; Excessively critical; Eyesight issues; Fiery; Headaches/migraines; Impatient with self and others; Indigestion/heartburn; Inflammation; Irritable; Judgmental; Mean; Skin rashes

Attached; Complacent; Congested—sinus and allergy problems; Dull; Greedy; Inert/immobile; Needy; Overeats when depressed; Overly protective; Overweight; Withdraws when sad or depressed

RHYTHMS OF AYURVEDA

Like all sentient creatures, we are designed to follow the laws of nature. First, our circadian rhythm follows the 24-hour day, moving from morning to afternoon to evening to night, with the sun and moon (depending on where you are) moving along from light to dark. We also have the lunar cycle of the moon, a monthly cycle, which governs the tidal cycle of the oceans. And finally, we have a seasonal rhythm, the 12-month yearly cycle. If we pay attention, we can notice how our bodies respond to the various cycles of day and night, the seasons, and even the phases of the moon.

In addition, Ayurveda has a daily doshic cycle that equally affects all of the doshas. The qualities associated with each dosha are prevalent during certain times of the day. These cycles are the same for all doshas, as follows:

Vata Time: 2 a.m.–6 a.m. and 2 p.m.–6 p.m.

Pitta Time: 10 a.m.–2 p.m. and 10 p.m.–2 a.m.

Kapha Time: 6 a.m.–10 a.m. and 6 p.m.–10 p.m.

With this in mind, here is an ideal daily routine based on the doshic cycle:

Kapha Time 6 a.m.–10 a.m.

- Wake up around 6 a.m., without an alarm.
- Preform your morning routine (see page 50).
- Exercise: Kapha time is a good time to get moving.
- Meditate facing east (toward the rising sun). At this time, the mind should feel alert and awake; it's perfect for meditation.
- Eat breakfast when you feel hungry.
- Begin your daily activities.

Pitta Time 10 a.m.–2 p.m.

- Eat the most nutrient-dense meal of the day (protein is best had at this time of day).
- Rest quietly for a few minutes and allow your food to digest.
- Take a short walk after eating to promote digestion.

Vata Time 2 p.m.–6 p.m.

- The good meal you had during Pitta time will give you plenty of energy that is supported by Vata to be creative, work hard, and perform daily chores.
- Meditate at dusk facing north for cooling, calming energy.

Kapha Time 6 p.m.–10 p.m.

- Begin to wind down, avoiding heavy mental chores.

- Have an easy-to-digest dinner.

- Take a walk. Read spiritual or enjoyable texts. Avoid violent or scary TV and movies.

- Do light, enjoyable activities that promote relaxation.

Pitta Time 10 p.m.–2 a.m.

- Perform your evening routine (see page 52).

- Be in bed by 10 p.m., as Pitta digestion time begins now.

- This is the time when the body begins the cycle of daily repair and renewal. This is a crucial time of day, as Pitta time works now to digest and transform everything you took in during the day, including all of your experiences, thoughts, emotions, and food. During this process, nutrients and waste are separated. Waste is prepared to be eliminated in the morning. Nutrients are assimilated to heal, repair, and detox the body.

Vata Time 2 a.m.–6 a.m.

- Our most vivid dreams occur once the body has completed the metabolic process.

- If we do not go to sleep before this time, the winds of Vata keep us awake—hence the term "second wind."

- If we wake during this time, it can be hard to fall back to sleep. Use a mantra (see page 110) and breath work (see page 115) to lull yourself back to sleep.

- Awakening before 6 a.m., you will feel the wind and movement of Vata encouraging you to begin your day. You may notice that sometimes you awaken naturally around 5 a.m. or 6 a.m. and feel wide awake. If you decide to go back to sleep, you may wake up at 7 a.m. or 8 a.m. feeling sluggish. This is because you have entered Kapha time. Be aware of the doshic cycle, and use it to your benefit.

- According to the elemental effects on the times of day, our bodies respond accordingly. However, we often fight against it. Make note of the 24-hour doshic cycle, and see how you can use it to promote balance and harmony in your life. It is better to work with it, rather than against it. The elements and the universe will support you!

Maintaining Balance

One Ayurvedic principle is that "like attracts like." We can be easily thrown off balance if we keep attracting the same things to us. That's why this system employs the law of opposites to help us create balance. Let's say you are feeling dull, heavy, slow, and sluggish. A meal of eggs with cheese and bacon, which is heavy, oily, and slow to digest will just make you feel more of the same. Instead, you would want to eat the opposite of what you are feeling, which would be something light and dry, perhaps puffed cereal with goat's milk or a bowl of beans cooked with detoxifying spices and a light oil, like sunflower oil. And, if you are feeling ungrounded, you would gravitate toward warm, cooked foods and spices such as oatmeal with ginger, cinnamon, and turmeric to ground you.

To help us understand the law of opposites, Ayurvedic texts provide us with a list of 20 common qualities, or attributes, that are experienced in varying degrees throughout nature. The idea is that too much, or too little, of any one quality can throw us off balance, so we would turn to its opposite for healing.

AYURVEDA'S 20 QUALITIES

Heavy — Light

Slow — Quick

Cold — Hot

Oily — Dry

Smooth — Rough

Solid — Liquid

Soft — Hard

Stable — Moving

Subtle — Large

Clear — Sticky

The law of opposites is a fairly easy-to-understand concept, but not all of the Ayurvedic concepts are so straightforward. Other concepts include the three universal qualities (*gunas*), as well as the five layers, or sheaths (*koshas*). While it's helpful to be at least a little familiar with them, you don't need to delve into it all just yet to start dipping your toes into the dietary recommendations and lifestyle practices found in this book. If you want to know more, I encourage you to turn to appendix B on page 158 for an overview. Later on, when you start to get into a good routine and begin feeling great, you may choose to further your studies of Ayurvedic concepts.

Mind-Body-Spirit

Before we go too deeply into the everyday practices of Ayurveda, it's important to understand the meaning of mind-body-spirit. Ayurveda teaches that what happens in the physical body is reflected in the mind and spirit, and vice versa. In other words, if the body is suffering from a physical ailment or imbalance, it will negatively affect the other two aspects. Looking at this somewhat vague term from an Ayurvedic perspective can shed some light on its meaning and how it relates to us. In Ayurveda, the mind-body-spirit can also be viewed as the three dimensions: subtle, gross, and causal.

- The subtle dimension is the mind (consciousness), the intellect (decision-making process), and the ego (power, position, possessions, self-image).

- The gross dimension is the physical body and the environment and the interaction with the environment, such as breathing.

- The causal dimension comprises the personal (soul, memories, and desires); collective (creative desires); and universal (beyond time and space as we know it, where we are all interconnected, one).

The takeaway here is that you need to be aware that whatever you put into your body, you are also feeding to your mind and spirit. And it works the other way, too. When you take care of one, all three benefit.

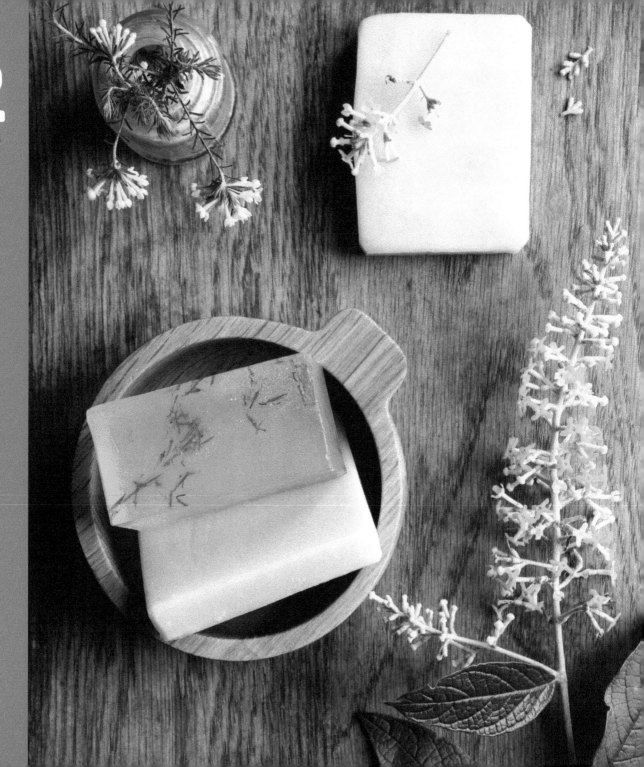

CHAPTER 2

The Path to Healing and Wellness

In Ayurveda, wellness is described as the absence of disease. When you are disease-free, you are healthy, vibrant, and at ease with yourself and others. When disease of mind or body is present, that vibrancy dissipates, and you are uncomfortable with yourself, and perhaps with others.

Ayurvedic healing involves customizing a treatment plan that addresses your needs as an individual. Once you have an idea of what your dosha is, and identify your chief concern (e.g., weight, menopause, anger, skin rashes, heartburn, depression, or anxiety), you can begin to create a daily routine that will support you in balancing yourself and addressing the areas where you feel out of balance. The first step, however, is figuring out what is *not* working in your life. What causes illness in the first place? Let's take a look.

THE SOURCE OF ILLNESS

In Ayurveda, good digestion is one of the keys to good health. When toxins, or *ama,* are minimal, your life essence, or *ojas,* can flow unimpeded in the circulatory channels. When ama is high, ojas is impeded, resulting in a host of issues. What this means is that when your body and mind are not taxed by accumulated toxins, everything in life flows more smoothly.

Ama is caused by low digestive "fire" (*agni*), which means your food is not being properly digested, the nutrients are not being assimilated, and waste is not being efficiently eliminated. (Other factors can lead to an excess of ama as well, which I'll discuss shortly.) This undigested food accumulates in the stomach and intestines where it can produce gas, bloating, candida overgrowth, and other toxins. It can squash the good bacteria, impeding your metabolic and digestive functions. If we do not move toxins out on a regular basis, we may find ourselves sick, or at least with a general feeling of malaise.

Ama can also be caused by environmental toxins (see page 20), and it can be caused by mental/spiritual anguish. Remember, what happens in the body on a physical level, can also affect us mentally and spiritually, and vice versa.

Signs of Ama in the System

- Chronic inflammation
- White, yellow, or dark coating on tongue (see page 83)
- Depression
- Difficulty making decisions
- Dull appetite
- Feeling foggy
- Gas, bloating, or heartburn
- Generalized pain and fatigue
- Getting sick often
- Incomplete or "messy" bowel movements
- Joint pain
- Scanty urine
- Sense of pessimism, detachment, impassivity
- Slow-healing wounds
- Sour or foul-smelling breath and body odor
- Weak immune system

Signs of Ojas Flowing in the System

- Body moves with ease regardless of weight
- Breath and body odor smell pleasant and clean
- Clear mind
- Elimination is smooth and regular
- Feeling rested upon awakening
- Focused and clear-headed throughout the day
- Healthy complexion
- Rarely getting sick
- Sense of enthusiasm, optimism, and excitement
- Strong digestion
- Uncoated tongue (see page 83)

As mentioned, when food is only partially digested, toxins accumulate in the body. This occurs when we eat before the previous meal has had time to fully digest; when we eat foods in the wrong combination (e.g., fruit and other foods); and when we eat processed foods, which are filled with preservatives, artificial colors, unnatural flavors, sugars, bulking agents, and so on.

When a chemical-laden food (e.g., Cheez Doodles) hits your system, I imagine the body goes through a thought process something like this: First it looks for the nutrients in the food. After an exhaustive search, it comes up empty and says, "Okay, what else is here that I can use?" Fake cheese flavor, really bad oil, and six different artificial food dyes, as well as a host of preservatives. So the body gives up and says, "Dude, there is nothing even remotely resembling food that I can use to build tissues, supply healthy fats, feed the brain, clean the blood—there is nothing here that is useful." So it gives up. That "food" becomes waste. It is sticky and heavy and sits in your body until it's finally forced out, probably in a very uncomfortable, messy bowel movement.

Toxins can also accumulate when we eat on the run; eat stale or leftover food, microwaved food, and frozen food; and eat while upset or standing up. There is an ancient Ayurvedic proverb that says if you eat while standing up, death is watching over your shoulder. The practical answer is that when you stand, you are not paying proper attention to the act of eating and what you are eating. So sit down in a comfortable setting with little distraction and pay attention and give thanks to your wonderful, healthy, "real" food.

With regard to toxins on a mental and emotional level, when you stew in your emotions and get caught up focusing on and thinking about things that are not going well in your life and in the outside world, you are creating ama—remember, what happens spiritually and mentally will also affect you physically. So think about areas of your life where you feel underserved, misunderstood, sad, and so on. Make a list of these "problems" and next to them, jot down a list of "solutions." By coming up with potential solutions, you are creating a path for ojas to flow. You may be surprised that the solution is easier than you thought.

For example, let's say that you feel that your spouse isn't contributing to the household chores. Here's a solution: Ask your spouse for support in a loving way, clearly and unemotionally laying out your case and your feelings. Together, create a plan to split the chores or look into getting a housekeeper, and be open to the resulting conversation without defensiveness or drama. If you chose to just stew in your emotions and imagine the conversation not going well in your head, you are creating ama. By speaking to your partner in a loving, open way, ojas can begin to flow. Wallowing in ama will eventually lead to feeling unwell (remember, what happens on any level affects the other levels), so it's best to recognize it as soon as possible, come up with a solution, and begin to let it go.

HOW TOXINS ACCUMULATE

Basically, toxins increase when we are not living in a healthy way and in harmony with nature. If you are not expressing yourself and hiding your emotions, toxins are having a field day. If you are staying up late watching scary (anxiety-provoking) movies, and thoughtlessly snacking on chips or ice cream, you probably have a lot of ama in your system. If you work on the computer or other screens up until bedtime, you are also increasing ama. If you don't get out into the sun or surround yourself in nature for at least 30 minutes a day, you are accumulating toxins (see Sun Gazing on page 124, and Earthing on page 122). If you do not eliminate properly in the morning—yup—you are holding on to toxins, so always follow your natural urges (see "Follow Natural Urges" on page 21).

Toxins in Everyday Life

It's not just the food we eat or the urges we suppress that introduce toxins to the body. We are surrounded by environmental toxins, too. If you live near conventional (nonorganic) farmland, you may be at risk of exposure to glyphosate and other herbicides and pesticides. So while the food you eat may be organic, the air you breathe isn't.

Follow Natural Urges

Ayurveda recommends not suppressing natural urges, which can cause a buildup of toxins in the mind and body. Here is a list of urges *not* to suppress:

- Belching
- Bowel movements
- Breathing heavily
- Coughing
- Crying
- Flatulence
- Hunger
- Orgasm, or suppression of genital fluids
- Sleeping
- Sneezing
- Thirst
- Urination
- Vomiting
- Yawning

Suppression of these urges can lead to disease. When "nature calls," attend to the matter at hand immediately. If not, as toxins build in the system, they can bury themselves deep into your tissues until a small problem that could have been easily corrected becomes a serious issue that might require drastic intervention. You can help yourself by letting go and expressing yourself on every level—including these natural urges.

Those in cities are exposed to high levels of toxic gases, fumes, and waste. The simple act of just *living* in our homes can expose us to chemicals in our furniture, carpets, paint, and even some hardwood and other types of flooring. So what's a person to do? Wrapping ourselves in organic cotton and breathing through a gas mask just isn't feasible, so how can we lessen the burden on the body?

Let's start by looking on our shelves and in the bathroom cabinet. I always ask my clients to tell me what cosmetics and body products they use, including shampoo and conditioner, deodorant, toothpaste, soap, moisturizer, nail polish, mascara, eye shadow, and hair dye.

One of the most popular brands of toothpastes has *seven* potentially toxic ingredients in it: triclosan, sodium lauryl sulfate (SLS), artificial sweeteners, fluoride, propylene glycol, diethanolamine (DEA), and microbeads (tiny plastic pellets that can penetrate the gums, not to mention go into the streams and waterways, and be eaten by fish, for which they prove toxic). This is why most toothpaste labels offer the warning "Do Not Swallow." They know that these ingredients, including fluoride, can be highly toxic when ingested. So why in the world would anyone put that in their mouth? There are several Ayurvedic companies like Auramere and Himalaya that make great, nontoxic toothpaste, but one of my favorite toothpastes is plain baking soda. You can even mix it with a little sea salt and turmeric for a spectacular way to clean your teeth. Add a few drops of organic peppermint or spearmint essential oil if you'd like.

Read the ingredients carefully on all of your body products and check them out on the website of the Environmental Working Group (www.ewg.org). The EWG rates many products that we use every day and can provide you with handy, easy-to-use information to help you make informed purchases. You can check out all your cosmetics for possible toxic chemicals at Campaign for Safe Cosmetics (www.safecosmetics.org).

Why is this so important? Because our bodies need to use energy wisely. If we are constantly gorging on bad food, slathering our bodies with hazardous chemicals, and coloring our hair with lethal dyes, our body spends all of its time just trying to alleviate the damage we are putting on it and in it. If we reduce the amount of toxins we use, then the body can use its precious energy to do what it's designed to do—repair tissues, clean the blood, assimilate nutrients, eliminate waste, and rejuvenate the mind, body, and spirit. If your energy is being wasted just trying to get rid of what you intentionally added, then you are not efficiently using your vehicle to help yourself move forward in the world and heal yourself and others.

Questions to Ask Yourself

On Your Body: Read the ingredients of everything you put *on* your body.

- What's in the brand of toothpaste you use?

- What's in the brand of deodorant you use?

- What's in the brand of shampoo/conditioner you use?

- What's in the brand of moisturizer you use?

- What's in the brand of shaving cream you use?

- What's in the brand of mascara you use?

- What's in the brand of lipstick or lip balm you use?

- What's in the brand of hair color, permanent, or straightening product you use?

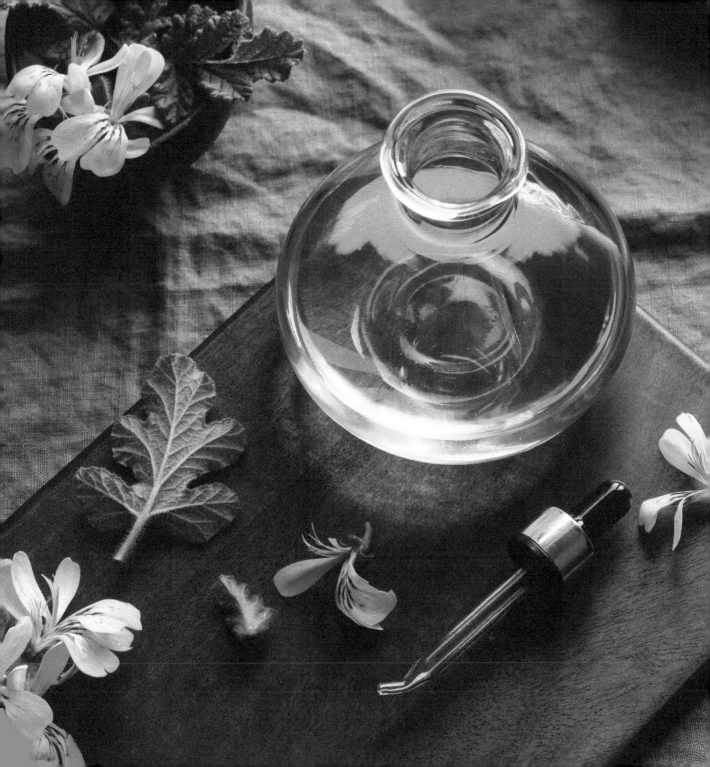

Look Before You Flush!

The quality and frequency of your bowel movements can tell you a lot about your current state of health. For each dosha, there are certain characteristics to look for. When your bowel movements are not normal, take steps to eliminate what is not working and to add in food and supplements that promote better digestion, along with more healthy and balancing practices into your lifestyle.

VATA BALANCED Elimination within two to three hours of waking; little to no odor; elimination feels complete; hard stool; dark brown; no gas

PITTA BALANCED Well-formed but soft; breaks up when flushing; mild odor; twice a day, usually upon waking and after a meal

KAPHA UNBALANCED Sticky, soft or "mushy"; mucus can be seen; need to wipe several times to clean; incomplete elimination

VATA UNBALANCED No daily bowel movement (or every few days); hard, dark balls; elimination doesn't feel complete; astringent odor; excessive gas

PITTA UNBALANCED Runny, yellowish, or greenish stool or diarrhea; more than twice a day; unpleasant odor; burning sensation

KAPHA BALANCED Regular elimination upon waking; once or twice a day; well-formed; brown; large quantity; little odor or even a sweet smell; clean wipe

- What's in the brand of nail polish you use?

- What's in the brand of body wash or bar soap you use?

In Your Home: Do the items you use to clean your home contain any chemicals? Go to the website of the Environmental Working Group (www.ewg.org) to check.

- What laundry detergent do you use?

- Do you use dryer sheets?

- What brand of dishwashing liquid do you use?

- How do you clean your floors?

- What type of duster do you use?

- What spray cleaners are you using in your house and bath?

- Do you change your dish sponge often?

In Your Mind: What you are putting into your head? Do the activities you are engaging in make you feel relaxed, or do they cause you to feel agitated, frightened, frustrated, or stressed out?

- What type of TV shows and movies do you watch? Do they make you feel good, or do they cause anxiety?

- Do you read scary or disturbing books, or books that enrich you with positive feelings?

- Do you take time to breathe deeply and walk around during the workday, or do you remain at your desk until your work is done?

- Do you work more than 40 hours a week, leaving little time for yourself?

- Do you set aside time for vacations?

- Do you give yourself time away from screens and monitors, or do you look at your smartphone or laptop until it is time for bed?

A TYPICAL AYURVEDIC CONSULTATION

As you are beginning your Ayurvedic practice, there is much you can do to heal on your own, as you'll discover in part 2. Once you start seeing how some simple practices help, you may want to know more and schedule a visit with an Ayurvedic practitioner. So what might happen at a typical visit?

Often, a person comes in complaining of one symptom or another as their chief concern—for example, excess weight, trouble sleeping at night, feeling stressed out, or constipation. After a few questions from the practitioner, it may become clear that their initial concern was actually just a symptom of something deeper. There is almost always something else going on that creates these states of imbalance, and this is good to know as you embark on your healing journey.

An Ayurvedic consultation uses many tools of detection and observation to discern what the real problem is. Through questions and interpretation of diagnostics tools—examinations of the tongue, skin, sense of smell, eyes, fingernails, and reading the pulses—a trained counselor can determine where you are out of balance and create a sustainable path to wellness. For example, a person complaining of headaches might also have heartburn and a skin rash, and are going prematurely bald or gray. They may also be defensive, impatient, straightforward, and intense.

A practitioner will see right away that this person has a Pitta imbalance (see the chart on page 10 for signs of imbalance for each of the doshas). And while addressing the headache symptoms may make the client feel better, what the practitioner is really doing is pacifying Pitta by recommending cooling foods, cooling pranayama (breath work like Cooling Breath, see page 117), and making other lifestyle recommendations.

In my case, I was at least 40 pounds overweight. I thought that was my problem. But I learned from an Ayurvedic practitioner that it was just a symptom of Kapha imbalance, and that weight loss was just a benefit to me reducing Kapha. Reducing Kapha physically can mean reducing dairy, wheat, and sugar in the diet. Mentally, it can mean letting go of old beliefs, routines, and patterns: throwing things away, creating space, and taking care of and nurturing oneself first.

For a primarily Vata person, complaints to their practitioner often have to do with digestion, gas, and bloating, which can be easily remedied by eating warm cooked foods, using good oils, and decreasing raw and cold foods. Other recommendations would include engaging in grounding and nurturing exercises like yoga and Tai Chi, or swimming in warm water. Dressing warmly and sticking to a schedule of eating can go a long way in balancing Vata.

So do you need an Ayurvedic practitioner to begin healing? Not necessarily. If you need more help further down the line, look for a good Ayurvedic practitioner in your area or ask for recommendations.

NURTURE YOURSELF FIRST

As they tell you on an airplane, put your oxygen mask on first, before helping others with theirs! If you don't, you'll start feeling light-headed very quickly, and you won't be much help to anyone else. Often, people begin to feel unwell because they spend too much time taking care of others, to the detriment of their own health. And they don't really notice it until they fall apart. This is true of both men and women, with each sex trying to fulfill their traditional roles (women as nurturers and keepers of the home front, and men as the money-makers and providers). Those traditional roles are rarely reflective of reality these days, but those old-fashioned expectations are persistent. Each partner in a relationship, regardless of the demands placed upon them, needs to be sure their own needs are being met. An Ayurvedic routine—a complete system of self-care—is an excellent beginning.

There are also many single people who are trying to make it all work on their own, including placing demands on themselves to find a life partner to feel fulfilled. It's only natural to want to partner with someone. That is the way our world is set up, and when the union is right, there is nothing better. But a single person—as I once was—can be equally fulfilled if they value their relationship with themselves enough to practice nurturing self-care. I wish I had a dollar for every person who has told me that they don't cook themselves meals because *it's just for them*! Who better to cook for, to care for, to nurture, than yourself?

If you recognize yourself in either scenario, Ayurveda guides you toward putting on your own oxygen mask first. It helps you unravel the conundrums and find your healing path. Ayurveda can help you clear the cobwebs in your mind away, and begin to see clearly that your perfect health and well-being is the key to the well-being of all people. There is a beautiful saying in Hebrew: *Tikkun olam*. It means "repair the world." But to repair the world, you must repair yourself. Ayurveda holds the key.

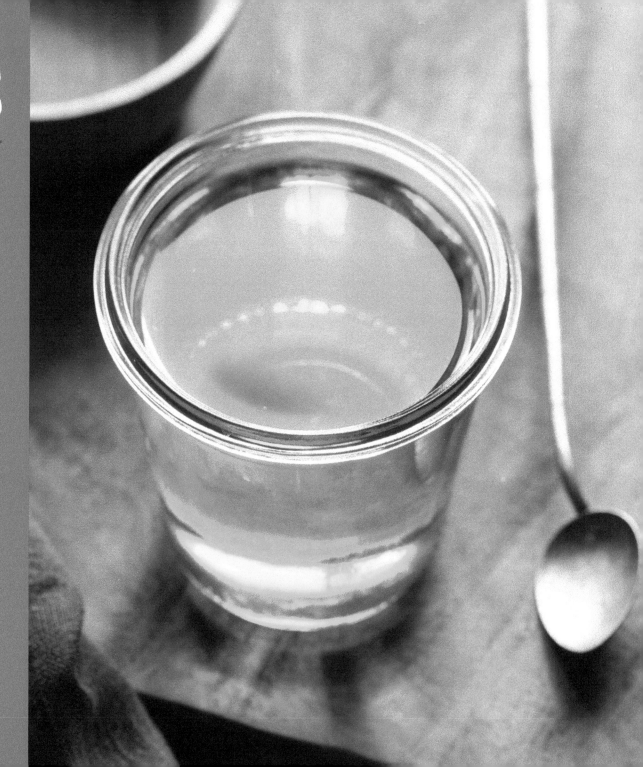

CHAPTER 3

An Overview of Ayurvedic Healing Methods

When Ayurvedic practitioners work on healing a doshic imbalance in their patients, they may, in addition to other recommendations and practices, prescribe certain herbs known for balancing the doshas. Depending on the individual's constitution, they can be delivered in the form of tablets or capsules, powders, or a simple mixture that can be licked off a spoon. And depending on the specific doshic imbalance, they may mix the herbal preparations with ghee, aloe, or milk.

But you don't need to know how to do this on your own. There are many ways you can begin to heal yourself with the basic Ayurvedic techniques and recipes discussed in part 2. Be prepared to make changes, but remember to take it slowly. Small changes can have profound effects. Let's start by looking at some of the basics, including dietary guidelines and other practices you may want to start trying.

BASIC DIETARY GUIDELINES

Ayurveda recommends avoiding certain foods that can create toxic residue in the body called ama. The foods to avoid include frozen meals, leftovers (over 36 hours max), processed foods, microwaved foods, and canned soups and sauces with lots of additives. All these foods have a diminished life force, or *prana*.

While it is important to reduce consumption of certain foods, it is just as important to increase and add in other foods, many of which are included in the recipes in chapter 5. Certain foods are easier to digest, so the body can use its energy for healing and repairing. Also, it is important to follow certain guidelines, such as reducing the consumption of cold foods in winter and hot foods in the summer (see chapter 8, which includes seasonal suggestions).

Some basic guidelines to try, which worked wonders for me, include the following:

- Begin your day with hot water and lemon or lime in the morning (see page 85).

- Sip warm water or tea throughout the day.

- Eat three meals a day. Do not snack between meals. After you eat, your body uses that food for energy and stores what is not needed at that time. Between meals, your body is able to dig deep to use stored pockets of energy to keep you going. Even if you munch on carrots or apple slices throughout the day, you are depriving your body of this natural period of detox—using what is already there. If you are hungry between meals, you are probably not eating enough nutrient-rich food at each meal. (On occasion, the timing may be that there is time for only two meals. That's okay, especially for Kapha who may actually do best with just two meals. There's more on this later.)

- Do not mix fruit with other foods. Eat fruit 45 minutes to one hour before any meal, ideally before breakfast. This is not considered snacking. When you wait that 45 minutes to an hour, your digestive juices will have plenty of time to process the nutrients in the fruit before your main meal.

- Do not eat raw salad veggies or cold fruit or drinks. Avoid ice. Raw food is difficult for the body to process, interfering with digestion. The same is true for cold food.

- Each meal should be about two open handfuls of food, which represents two-thirds of your stomach. (A person with larger hands generally has a larger stomach.) In other words, eat until you are 80 percent full, leaving 20 percent space for the digestive "fires" to metabolize your food.

- Do not overeat. You should feel energized after eating, not wiped out and stuffed. If you feel that way, you ate too much or combined food in a way that made it hard to digest. It's like putting too many logs on the fire—it smothers the flame. Eat just enough to keep your digestion burning bright! Two handfuls—like a large bowl—should be plenty, if the food you choose is nutrient rich and easy to digest.

- Eat less protein than is typical in a Western diet. In the evening, eat only light amounts of protein, or none at all. Unless you are working the nightshift, in which case your daily cycle is not the norm, you are probably consuming more protein than you need with dinner.

- Don't mix proteins. A buffet can be very confusing with all the offerings. Even if you pile on the "good" foods like beans, tofu, eggs, cottage cheese, and lean meats, you are taxing the body. Each protein digests at a different rate, so stick to one protein per meal.

- Make lunch your most important meal of the day. It should be densely packed with nutrients, including protein and carbohydrates. This meal is often consumed during work hours, but it is very important to pay attention while

When you burp, that is your indication that you have eaten enough food, regardless of what's left on your plate or in your bowl. There has been many a meal that I belched just about when I thought I was only halfway through—and there it was. Even one more mouthful will set you over the line of feeling good to feeling stuffed. So you think you don't burp? Pay attention, because I promise that you do. Your stomach knows when it's about two-thirds full and it lets you know by pushing the air out. So push the plate away, and enjoy the feeling of eating until just satisfied.

you eat. Turn away from the computer, and sit outside if possible.

- Make dinner the easiest-to-digest meal of the day. Easy-to-digest foods include light proteins (if you must have protein with your dinner) such as fish, warm and cooked foods, soups, and sautéed greens (which interestingly have a calming effect). Eat dinner at least three hours before bed.

- Breakfast, while not as important as the most substantial meal of the day between 10 a.m. and 2 p.m., is important, primarily for Pitta and Vata. For these types, it should be warm, nourishing, and easy to digest. Kapha may simply enjoy a bowl of fruit or a light grain porridge.

- Always sit to eat your meals. In general, it is very important to take the time to sit down when eating to be fully present at your meal. Sit and enjoy the process of eating and noticing what is on your plate. Sitting in your car to eat doesn't count.

- Walk after meals. Taking a short walk after lunch and dinner will encourage digestion.

- Sleep on your left side. This will help promote digestion. When you sleep on your left side, your major organs are supported and your digestive juices flow naturally.

You might not be able to make huge shifts and do everything on this list, but even something as simple as avoiding cold water and sipping warm water throughout the day can have a profound effect on the body. The healing benefits of eating at least two to three meals a day (which might be more or less than you are used to), not snacking between meals, and having a light dinner at least three hours before bed can make an enormous difference in your health and well-being. Eating this way allows your body to work most efficiently, stoking your digestive "fires" at meals and digesting your food properly, giving it time to work on detoxing and repairing tissues between meals.

Trying some of these dietary guidelines for a few weeks can shift your awareness to a higher level, preparing you to make further changes and delve more deeply into an Ayurvedic lifestyle. You'll have a chance to start a 21-day routine in chapter 4, and then it's up to you if you want to take this new, health-enhancing lifestyle even further. Here are a few more recommendations to help you make the shift:

- If you are a coffee drinker, add a pod of cardamom to your unground coffee beans before grinding them, or a pinch of ground cardamom to your brewed coffee. This spice reduces the acid in the coffee, making it easier on the stomach.

- Eat ghee daily. To learn more about this amazing oil, see All About Ghee on page 33. Incidentally, do not combine equal parts ghee and honey in a meal, as this can increase toxins in the body. The ancient texts strongly advise against doing this, so please don't try it!

- Begin your day with the Ayurvedic jam *chyawanprash*. Chyawanprash has many ingredients that work together to promote optimal health by rejuvenating the tissues and strengthening many functions of the

All About Ghee

Ghee is clarified butter. You'll find a recipe to make this delicious golden elixir on page 58, but it may also be available for purchase in your grocery store (buy only organic). Ghee is used in many Ayurvedic medical treatments. It comes from the cow, which is considered sacred in India. Practically, it is one of the best systems to deliver nutrients deep down into all seven layers of your tissues (plasma, blood, muscle, fat, bone, nervous system, and reproductive tissues in both men and women). So cooking with ghee is essential to good overall health— use more for Vata and Pitta and a little less for Kapha.

You may think that because ghee comes from dairy, its high fat content couldn't possibly be healthy, but let me assure you that ghee has many healing qualities. After just three months of eating ghee daily, I lost 30 pounds. If I may, allow me to sing the praises of ghee:

HIGH-HEAT COOKING OIL has a higher smoking point than olive oil and coconut oil

GREAT FOR SAUTÉING spices to bring out their healing qualities

KEEPS FOR MONTHS, EVEN YEARS, at room temperature, as long as it does not get wet

FULL OF MEDIUM-CHAIN FATTY ACIDS, which are easily absorbed by the body and burned as energy

RICH IN BUTYRIC ACID, a short-chain fatty acid, which promotes a healthy digestive tract

CAN BE USED BY ALL DOSHAS but is most beneficial to Vata because it has all the qualities that Vata needs to help lubricate, warm, and strengthen; they should slather it on everything, including their bodies! Kapha does best with moderate use. Very balancing for Pitta.

DECREASES CHOLESTEROL and triglyceride levels when used properly

body. A tablespoon of chyawanprash every morning, licked off the spoon while sipping hot water, can benefit everyone. (There are several brands you can purchase; see the resources on page 161.)

- End your day by drinking Golden Milk (see page 60) and taking triphala, a toner for the bowels, and the most widely used Ayurvedic supplement (see page 144). Available in tablets and powder, triphala is made from three detoxifying and tonifying fruits that help you more effectively absorb and assimilate nutrients and get rid of waste through healthy bowel movements. Two tablets should be about right, but an Ayurvedic practitioner may prescribe more or less to maintain health.

- If you like a glass of wine or beer, knowing which dosha you are can help you make a good choice: Vata does best with sweet wines, Pitta does best with beer, and Kapha does best with dry wines. None of the doshas do well with hard alcohol unless it is prescribed by an Ayurvedic practitioner. Ayurvedic concoctions called *arishtams* or *kashayams* are highly effective fermented medicines, but they should be used only under guidance.

Using Tastes to Guide Food Choices

In Ayurveda, we divide food into six categories: sweet, sour, salty, pungent, bitter, and astringent. Each taste corresponds to a dosha, and more or less of it can either create balance or imbalance. But we do want some representation of all six tastes in every meal, as that is the most satisfying way to eat. Ayurvedic guidelines aren't intended to make you feel deprived or left out.

The Western diet is composed mostly of sweet, sour, and salty. It's no wonder that we have an obesity epidemic, that irritable bowel syndrome and disorders are prevalent, and many other diseases abound, as these are the heaviest, most addictive foods. When we solely eat from these categories, our bodies have no chance to heal and repair. To help us create balance in the mind and body, it is imperative that we include food from the pungent, bitter, and astringent categories. These three tastes effectively wring out excess toxins from the body.

Interestingly, the word *rasa* in Sanskrit can mean both taste and emotion. So there is really no such thing as non-emotional eating. It's all tied together—mind and body. Ayurveda also teaches why sweet is the most satisfying of tastes—it's the first thing we taste: Mother's milk, which is naturally sweet. We all crave different tastes at different times, and it's almost always tied to an emotion. A fascinating exploration in Ayurveda leads us to understand why we crave or desire certain foods. Let's break it down by taste:

SWEET

Sweet foods are the most satisfying of all the tastes, and they are tied to intensely satisfying emotions as well. Sweet foods, in appropriate amounts, can create feelings of deep emotional ties, love and compassion, satisfaction, and a sense of caring and being cared for. When taken in excess, sweetness can promote inertia, dullness, and neediness.

Notice how you feel when you just have a bite or two of something sweet, and how it feels when you eat the whole cake. Ask yourself: "What is it I need? Maybe a hug? Perhaps I need to love more, or allow myself to be loved?" I advise my clients who have intense sweet cravings to look for new outlets to express their own sweetness. Maybe volunteer at a dog shelter, help out an elderly relative or neighbor, do random acts of kindness, add money to parking meters, pay the toll for the person in the car behind you, or be kind to yourself. All of these actions really can lessen the physical craving for something sweet.

What are sweet foods? Sweet is the most densely nutritive of tastes and includes proteins, carbohydrates, fats, grains, dairy, breads, pasta, starchy vegetables, sweet fruits, nuts, oils, sugar, honey, and all animal products, including meat, chicken, and fish.

Vata and Pitta both benefit from sweet foods, as they need more water and grounding, and sweetness. Kapha, who is made of the sweet elements of earth and water, should take sweet in moderation, and perhaps avoid it completely during times of too much Kapha.

SOUR

Sour foods, when eaten in moderation, can stimulate appetite and digestion, and feel warming and refreshing. In excess, sour foods can feel heavy and hot, and emotions can be negative, pessimistic, and irritable. When a person craves sour foods, they might take a look at how they are viewing the world. Is it you against them? Do you place blame on others and cry "sour grapes" when things don't go your way? Stepping back and assessing the situation can help the "sour" person gain perspective. Cooling off and drying out a bit by eating fewer sour foods and taking a fresh look at the world, situations, and people around you can help balance the sour emotion.

What are sour foods? They are refreshing, acidic, and sparkly: Citrus fruits, sour fruits, tomatoes, yogurt, cheese, pickles, most vinegars, and some alcohol.

Vata benefits from eating sour as it comprises the elements of earth and fire, which Vata lacks. Pitta and Kapha will be aggravated by sour. It's too hot for Pitta, and too wet for Kapha.

SALTY

Salty promotes digestion and, when used in moderation, enhances the flavor of most foods. Emotionally, a balanced "salty behavior" can help you be more outspoken and address your needs and desires. If you have too much salt, it can lead to feelings of greediness and addiction (try eating just a few kernels of salted popcorn, chips, or French fries—it's hard). Salty personality traits include feeling angry, grouchy, and irritated. If you find yourself craving salt, take a look at your life and see where you may not be expressing yourself. Perhaps you need to speak up more often and express your needs in a balanced way.

Salty foods include seafood, seaweed, some meat, salt, and snacks. Check the labels of canned and frozen foods, as they may contain excess salt.

Vata benefits from the water and fire elements of salt. Pitta and Kapha, hot and wet respectively, are aggravated by the salty taste.

PUNGENT

Pungent taste detoxifies, stimulates digestion, and is heating and drying. Emotionally, when taken in small amounts, pungent food can create clarity, purpose, and motivation. It can act to cut through heaviness or fogginess. Too much can promote abrasiveness, anger, and aggression. If you crave pungent foods, you may be looking for a way to express pent-up anger or frustration. Be careful not to "blow up" from too much fire. Look for ways to cool down—take a swim or walk in the evening or early morning when it's cool. Drink some coconut water. Examine the areas in your life where you feel trampled upon, and choose to move aside and rise up with grace.

Foods that contain the pungent taste include ginger, hot peppers, tomato salsa, cloves, thyme, basil, cayenne pepper, radishes, mustard, wasabi, chili peppers, garlic, and onions.

Kapha should adore pungent foods as they balance their cold, wet nature and it can help them shed extra weight. Pungent, comprising the elements of fire and air, should be limited by Pitta (heat) and Vata (dry).

BITTER

Bitter foods are extremely detoxifying and can reduce inflammation. They are drying and cold, and can be very flavorful. A small amount of bitter can help clear the cobwebs and allow one to see things more clearly. Too much bitter can create a sense of grief and disillusionment. The bitter person is jealous, jaded, and mean. They hold grudges and blame others when things go wrong. When I have clients who feel bitter, they are usually holding on to things that no longer exist or are wishing for a different outcome that will never happen. Visualizing the world as it is, and situations exactly as they are, and learning to accept them can help alleviate feelings of bitterness. Knowing that you are holding it in, and that it's only damaging you, is key to understanding and letting go. Try new things in life. Collect new experiences. Let go of the past.

Foods containing the bitter taste include Swedish bitters (an herbal tonic that is added to juice or water); sorrel and other leafy greens; yellow vegetables; bitter herbs like chamomile, mint, and dandelion; and horseradish.

Bitter is good for Kapha, who often exudes sweetness and kindness (they can use a touch of bitter to balance these qualities). The cool, lightness of bitter can be balancing for Pitta. Vata should avoid large quantities of bitter for those same reasons; cool and light will increase Vata.

ASTRINGENT

Astringent foods are detoxifying and have a way of cleansing the palate—emotionally clearing the slate, allowing space to clear the mind and get back to work without any lingering emotions. Too much astringent, because it is so compacting, can lead to a loss of interest in activities and routines. A small amount goes a long way. Astringent is not very common but can be found in beans, lentils, pomegranates, cranberries, unripened bananas, black tea, and dark greens. People with an astringent emotional quality are often filled with bitterness as well. They look contracted, depleted, and dried out. It's hard for them to smile. The remedy is to add all the qualities of sweet, sour, and salty—in abundance—into their lives. Guided meditation and sweet, floral, and spicy essential oils used daily can help. Getting out into the elements, including walking in the rain, and exposure to early-morning and evening sun, can do wonders.

In a nutshell, Vata benefits from sweet, sour, and salty. Pitta benefits from sweet, bitter, and astringent. And Kapha benefits from pungent, bitter, and astringent. Speaking of nuts, they are considered sweet, but they are very hot, making them best for Vata. Pitta and Kapha will want to avoid nuts, but most seeds are great for these two doshas.

Starting an Ayurvedic Kitchen

To start your Ayurvedic kitchen, you won't need to do a complete overhaul—just begin to make shelf and refrigerator space by using up what you have and replacing it with items that will serve you better. You'll find some basic guidelines in chapter 4 for preparing your kitchen. Meanwhile, in chapter 5, you will find some amazing recipes, which may include several ingredients you have never heard of before or are only slightly familiar with. Most of these are spices.

In appendix A on page 153, you will find a list of common Ayurvedic cooking ingredients, which can give you a heads-up on some of the ingredients you'll need to make the recipes. However, before you go out and purchase all of the items mentioned, choose your recipes, see what you need, and begin to make your grocery store purchases as needed.

DAILY PRACTICES AND BODYWORK

The Ayurvedic practices listed here are varied and many. Don't feel as if you need to incorporate them all into your daily routine. Even if you just include one or two, you will begin to feel better. Ayurveda is amazing in that way— subtle changes can have profound effects. Your body will respond because it has been waiting for this! In part 2, you will find a description of how to perform each practice and learn about the benefits of each.

- Aromatherapy (see page 90)
- Breath work (see page 115)
- Dry brushing (see page 86)
- Foot washing and oil massage (see page 125)
- Head oiling (see page 126)
- Meditation (see page 119)
- Nasya oil (see page 89)
- Neti pot (see page 88)
- Oil massage (see page 86)
- Oil pulling (see page 84)
- Sun gazing (see page 124)
- Tongue scraping (see page 83)
- Yoga (see page 92)

DOSHA-SPECIFIC GUIDANCE

Like attracts like. It's a law of the universe. Try to be aware of including food and activities in your day that will satisfy all three doshas, keeping in mind how you are feeling, the weather, your schedule, and which dosha might be aggravated (revealed by signs of imbalance; see page 10). On any given day, we may feel frustrated and angry (too much Pitta), or we may feel like pulling the covers over our head and not getting out of bed (too much Kapha), or we might be running late for a meeting because we were distracted by so many other things along the way (too much Vata). In Ayurveda, when discussing dosha imbalances, we are always talking about having too much of a doshic quality, not too little.

It's most important when practicing Ayurveda to be aware of your state of being every day. Some people may have an underlying illness or a persistent imbalance that must be constantly pacified, but everyone can change day to day. Stay aware, know yourself, and use the methods in this book to heal yourself subtly, 24 hours a day. That is really what Ayurveda is all about: allowing your body to naturally detox, 24 hours a day, by feeding and caring for yourself in ways that allow the body to easily do the work it was designed to do.

All of the doshas can be balanced with food, drink, exercise, meditation, breath work, and more. As mentioned earlier, each dosha is balanced by eating a combination of all six food categories, but you should limit or favor certain tastes in each meal depending on your needs. Exercise for each dosha is generally a combination of stretching (yoga), aerobics, and weights, with each activity designed to balance the doshas.

Meditation can be a challenge for some, and a salvation for others. Nevertheless, it is recommended for each dosha, with time and techniques to help you receive the most benefit. The doshas will also greatly benefit from learning breath work and exercises to enhance or calm imbalances. Chanting a mantra can help calm your thoughts, excite the mind, and open creative and healing channels. (All of these practices are explained in part 2.)

Vata Guidelines

Some of the qualities of Vata are cold, dry, rough, and ungrounded. So we choose to eat, exercise, and breathe in ways that mitigate or reduce those qualities. Vata should eat warm, cooked, easy-to-digest foods so that the body can conserve its energy to keep warm and healthy. Vata needs the energy used to digest raw food for other metabolic processes, including repairing the tissues and cleaning the blood. It's also important for Vata to create a schedule and try to stick to a routine—especially with meals. Vata is the only dosha who forgets to eat. They will eat half a candy bar and put the rest in their bag and forget it's there. This would never happen with Pitta or Kapha! In addition, because of Vata's natural inclination toward fear and worry, it's important for Vata to feel safe and secure.

- Food should be well-cooked and easy to digest, and eating should be accompanied by sipping warm liquid throughout the meal, preferably warm water.

- Favor sweet, sour, and salty tastes, which help nourish Vata.

- Reduce pungent, bitter, and astringent tastes, which increase Vata.

- Dress to stay warm. Wear layers even in summer. Wear a scarf in fall, winter, and early spring.

- Ideal exercises for Vata include grounding and slower-paced exercises, such as Tai Chi or Qigong; swimming in warm water; slow, gentle yoga; walking outdoors in warm weather; short hikes; and light bicycling on level ground.

Pitta Guidelines

Pitta attributes include hot, sour, and pungent, so we look to the opposites to balance this fire dosha. Pitta will gravitate toward those things that increase the dosha, as it thrives on hot, vibrant qualities. But when Pitta is out of balance, it can be damaging to oneself and others. Pitta loves spicy food and loves to tell you about it! They will sweat profusely when eating hot chiles and tell you how much they love it. But they will suffer later with heartburn or indigestion. So it's important to calm Pitta with sweet, cooling foods and to encourage less competition and challenges, and more cooperation in either solitary or team sports and activities.

- Favor cool food and drink. Pitta loves cold drinks, so gradually move from iced to chilled to cool to room temperature, if possible.

- Favor sweet, bitter, and astringent tastes, which balance the fiery qualities of Pitta.

- Reduce sour, salty, and pungent tastes, which increase Pitta.

- Avoid overheating when exercising.

- Ideal exercises for Pitta include medium-paced exercises, such as brisk walking or light jogging; swimming in cool water; non-competitive biking; cross-country skiing; and outdoor activities in cool weather.

Kapha Guidelines

Kapha, made of earth and water, is heavier and sturdier than the other doshas. If left to their own volition, they would eat sweet or heavy, oily, fried foods all day long. Creamy is another favorite texture of Kapha. But that just contributes to that heavy, dull, inert energy. The tastes of pungent, bitter, and astringent actually act to wring out excess Kapha in the body by drying it up and moving it out. Kapha often has a dull appetite, but if the clock reads 8 a.m. or 12 p.m. or 6 p.m., it *must* be time for a meal! So they will eat. If Kapha wants to lose weight, they can greatly benefit by having two meals a day. A large meal between 10 a.m. and 2 p.m. and a light meal in the late afternoon or early evening (5 p.m. or 6 p.m.) can be sufficient and can help in reducing excess Kapha.

- Favor a lighter diet of foods that are easy to digest, as Kapha tends to have sluggish digestion.

- Reduce dairy products, because they are cold, sweet, and sour, which are Kapha characteristics.

- Favor warm food and drink, as Kapha is generally cold. Chilled drinks and food increase Kapha, and one needs to expend a lot of energy to create warmth, which could be used for other metabolic processes.

- Do not drink copious amounts of water, as it increases Kapha. Just sip warm water throughout the day.

- Eat more pungent, bitter, and astringent tastes, as they wring out excess Kapha from the body.

- Reduce sweet, sour, and salty tastes, so as not to increase these qualities in sweet Kapha, which can cause weight gain and immobility.

- Dress to stay warm so your body can use its energy to rejuvenate and repair the body.

- Ideal exercises for Kapha include vigorous activities and long workouts that promote sweating such as running, aerobics, dance, rowing, active yoga, and weight training.

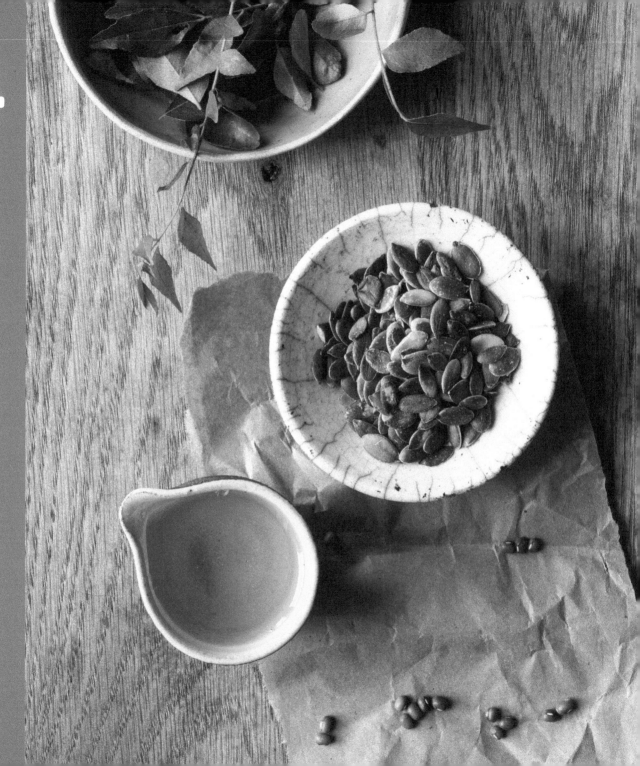

CHAPTER 4

A Gentle 21-Day Introduction to Ayurveda

When trying on anything new, remember to give yourself time and permission to be flexible. Hopefully you will have a lifetime to work these things into your daily practice, so take it one step at a time. Once you begin to see the benefits of Ayurveda, you will likely want to make this a permanent lifestyle, so begin slowly, learn the reasons behind the rituals, and see what makes you feel better. This is an individualized path, so you should take your time, move at your own pace, and add in new elements of Ayurveda when you feel ready. If you move slowly, you are more likely to stick with it.

There's no need to adopt this lifestyle all at once, or commit to it for several months or longer. You can simply dip your toes in for three weeks, using this chapter as your road map. Remember, you can do this on your own, but if you feel it would be helpful to you, go ahead and make an appointment with an Ayurvedic practitioner for further support.

3 STEPS TO BEGINNING AYURVEDA

Let's take a look at how to prepare the way for your new Ayurvedic lifestyle. First, be certain that this is a good time in your life to begin a transformational project. For example, if you are planning to go on vacation next week or if you are in the middle of a move, you may have difficulty committing to the 21-day plan. If you decide the time is right, begin to formulate your plan using a journal specifically for this purpose—your Ayurvedic journal.

1. Look at Your Current Condition

Define your chief concerns, or the main things in your life you want to change. Take a moment to sit quietly, breathe, and ask yourself the following questions—and remember, the Buddha said, "First thought, best thought." In other words, don't censor yourself. Let it flow. Answer the following questions in your Ayurvedic journal:

- What is not serving me in my life?

- If I could do anything I wanted to, what would it be?

- What is stopping me from moving forward?

Next, make a list of obstacles that may be interfering with your well-being, or problems currently at play in your life. Next to each one, jot down a simple solution. Don't worry about how the solution could happen, just write it down. For example:

Problem: At the end of the workday, I don't have the energy to cook a healthy meal.

Solution: Prep your ingredients for your evening meal in the morning so that everything is ready to go when it's time to cook dinner.

Problem: I don't know how to cook.

Solution: Take a cooking class and learn one recipe. Have a friend over to cook with you.

Problem: I don't have time in the mornings to spend doing a routine.

Solution: Wake up 10 minutes earlier and incorporate just one new practice. Don't hit the snooze button. Just get up!

2. Set Your Intention

Think about what you hope to gain by making changes in your life. Most assuredly, these will be positive things, so you will want to set an intention to make those things happen. Spend some quiet time thinking about this first. Then write down whatever occurs to you in your Ayurvedic journal. There's no need to write pages and pages; just a few thoughts or sentences can be enough to set your intention. Be sure to be specific in your needs and desires. And be positive! Once you've written it down, it will feel much more real.

3. Prepare Your Home

Set aside time to go through your home to determine what's not serving you. Start in your kitchen. Look in the cabinets, the refrigerator, and the freezer. Do you have junk food, processed foods, frozen entrées, and other less-than-healthy foods on hand? If so, maybe box up the nonperishables for another time or consider donating them. Finish up any perishables, but be sure to toss old leftovers into the trash or compost bin.

While you're in the kitchen, check to make sure you have some essential cookware. You don't want to cook with anything that has a Teflon coating, as Teflon can be toxic when scratched or overheated. You'll need a variety of pots and pans, but start with at least a 4-quart soup pot, one large pan, and one small pan. Some items that are helpful to have include an immersion blender, a countertop blender, a pressure cooker, a fine-mesh strainer, and a juicer. If you don't have these items, you don't have to run out to purchase them. Spend that money on your Ayurvedic-friendly supplies instead.

Next, take a look at the items in your bathroom, on your vanity, and in your cleaning-supply cabinet. Anything that contains harsh chemicals is not conducive to an Ayurvedic practice. You don't need to toss everything in the garbage, but do be aware of what you are running low on and make a plan to choose their healthier counterparts in the future.

If you can afford to, buy some Ayurvedic-friendly items. A few of my favorite brands of natural body products include Himalaya, Auramere, Dr. Bronner's, and JĀSÖN. And for home-cleaning products I especially like Seventh Generation. (You can also make your own multisurface cleaner with white vinegar, lemon juice, borax, and baking soda.) See the resources on page 161 for my recommendations.

YOUR 21-DAY AYURVEDIC SELF-CARE PLAN

Think in terms of weeks, rather than days. Week One will begin by getting your supplies together, learning a few recipes, and thinking about how you can begin implementing your daily routine, called *dinacharya*. Week Two will have you applying more Ayurvedic rituals into your day and more Ayurvedic meals into your plan. By week 3, you may find yourself inspired to keep learning new recipes, creating space and time for your morning routine, and beginning to implement your evening routine, which is part of your dinacharya.

Each week in the 21-Day Plan is divided into mind, body, and spirit. The following entries provide guidance on how you can nurture those parts of yourself. On page 48, you will find a worksheet you can use to create your own customized daily practices.

Week One

Mind: Focus on the changes you would like to see occur, and visualize the steps it will take to make them happen. In your Ayurvedic journal, write one step you will take each day to move toward feeling more balanced. List one thing that you can do for yourself to make you feel good, and list one thing you can let go of that no longer serves you. In addition, commit each day to work on making this happen, or at least to set a plan in motion.

Body: Prepare for the week by reading through the recipes in chapter 5. Choose three new recipes to try, making sure Kitchari is among them (see pages 61–66). You can have kitchari for any meal of the day. Make a pot of Everyday CCF Tea (see page 57) each morning and sip it throughout the day. Alternatively, you can prepare ginger tea by adding a few slices of fresh ginger to hot water. Sip it throughout the day.

Purchase a tongue scraper (see page 83), a dry brush (see page 86), nasya oil (see page 89), and abhyanga oil (see page 86) for the purposes of beginning your daily routine. Organic sesame seed oil is good to have on hand for oil pulling and other practices (not toasted sesame seed oil, which is only used in cooking!).

Spirit: Set up a time and space to meditate (see page 119) and do your breath work (see page 115) for at least five minutes. Download a supportive app on your smartphone or tablet, such as Insight Timer or Headspace. Log your meditation time in your Ayurveda journal or on your app. Increase the time by a few minutes each day throughout the week. Notice how you feel, and jot down a few words after you meditate to remind yourself of any insights or observations.

Week Two

Mind: Notice your feelings during this 21-day process. Do you feel resistance, acceptance, excitement, boredom, or something else? Whatever it is, write it down in your Ayurveda journal. Let all these emotions come up and out, and focus on what is making you feel better. If you find yourself creating obstacles on your path, write them down, ball them up, throw them away, and get back on the plan. Remind yourself that you are not your thoughts. Give yourself a pep talk. And remember baby steps—one thing at a time. There's no need to create blockages to making a few simple changes. Let it go, and come back to your enthusiasm.

Body: Review the sample routine on page 50, and begin your daily routine (dinacharya). Set out your tongue scraper, abhyanga oil, and dry brush. Make time in the mornings to put each practice into your morning routine. Make two new recipes this week. Find new breakfast foods you like among the recipes in chapter 5. Learn to make ghee (see page 58).

Spirit: Practice silent walking meditation outside in the elements. Notice how your body feels outside: moving, breathing, being connected. Immerse yourself in the elements. Practice Sun Gazing (see page 124) at dawn and dusk. Continue your meditation and breath work from the week before, extending the time a few minutes each day as you did in week one.

Week Three

Mind: Check in with yourself to see what is working and what is not working. Allow yourself to make adjustments until it feels right. Do not force anything. There's no need to be rigid. Go easy on yourself and allow change to take place naturally, at a slow pace.

Body: Every day or two, create a new meal. Pay attention to the seasons and learn which fruits and vegetables are in season, and when shopping, choose those fruits and vegetables. Make smaller portions of your meals to avoid having leftovers. (See the seasonal suggestions in chapter 8.)

Practice yoga every day for at least 10 minutes. Choose a few poses from chapter 6 that feel good to you, and work through them. If you can, sign up for a yoga class with a good teacher. Just once a week for a class is fine, but continue your daily yoga practice at home.

Start incorporating your evening routine into your dinacharya (see page 52). Oil your feet and scalp (see pages 125–126). Before bed, take triphala (see page 143) and drink Golden Milk (see page 60).

Spirit: Lengthen your meditation time, working toward 30 minutes a day. Be easy on yourself and others. Lower your expectations and accept things as they are, but with a vision of how they could be. Begin to practice self-inquiry meditation (see page 119) and continue your breath work.

Your Custom
Self-Care Plan Worksheet

With the guidance you've received in this chapter, use the following worksheet to create your own customized Ayurvedic daily practices.

WEEK 1							
	Sun	Mon	Tue	Wed	Thu	Fri	Sat
MIND							
BODY							
SPIRIT							
NOTES							

WEEK 2

	Sun	Mon	Tue	Wed	Thu	Fri	Sat
MIND							
BODY							
SPIRIT							
NOTES							

WEEK 3

	Sun	Mon	Tue	Wed	Thu	Fri	Sat
MIND							
BODY							
SPIRIT							
NOTES							

SAMPLE DAILY ROUTINE (DINACHARYA)

As mentioned earlier, in Ayurveda, we call our daily routine dinacharya. I have a pretty standard routine, but it changes according to the season, the amount of time I have, and how I'm feeling that day. Dinacharya will look a little different for everyone, but let's see one example of what a typical Ayurvedic-style day looks like.

Morning

- Wake up sometime between 6 a.m. and 7 a.m., preferably without an alarm. Sleeping with the shades open, if appropriate for your living situation, is a wonderful way to allow natural light to wake you up.

- Before getting out of bed, set your intention for the day. Take a few deep breaths into your belly and focus on what is important for you on this day. Take a moment to express gratitude, and name one thing that you will do just for yourself today.

- Sit up in bed. Do some gentle twisting and stretching to get your blood flowing. Stand and allow yourself to do a few Forward Bends (see page 101), inhaling up and exhaling down. Feel your heart beating. Give thanks.

- Move to the bathroom and take your time for complete elimination of the waste that was separated from the nutrients during the night. Urinate and give yourself time for a complete bowel movement. A Squatty Potty—a stool that fits around the toilet bowl on which you can rest your feet—is a great investment. You can use it to raise your knees to just above your hips to promote an easier bowel movement. Don't strain. Breathe deeply. The bowels evacuate best on the out breath. Relax. Notice the quality of your bowel movement (see page 24), as this is a clear indication of your health.

- After washing your hands, scrape your tongue with a tongue scraper or spoon. Notice if there is a coating on your tongue and what color it is (see page 83).

- Brush your teeth with a natural or Ayurvedic toothpaste (see brands I love on page 22) or with baking soda.

- Do oil pulling with either coconut oil or sesame seed oil (see page 84). Spit the oil into a trash can after 10 to 20 minutes. Do *not* spit the oil in the sink; it will clog your pipes.

- Rinse your mouth with ¼ teaspoon of baking soda mixed into some warm water.

- Drink a small glass of warm water with lemon or lime (see page 85). Do not drink your warm water until you have cleaned the bacteria out of your mouth, or you will just be ingesting what your body worked hard to expel during the night.

- If you live in a humid climate, have seasonal allergies, or are doing a cleanse, use a neti pot (see page 88).

- If you did not use a neti pot, use nasya oil in your nostrils (see page 89). If you did use a neti pot, wait at least one hour before applying oil to the nasal passages.

- Meditate for 20 to 30 minutes (see page 119).

- Exercise appropriately for your dosha. Ayurveda encourages exercising during Kapha time of day, so it's best anytime between 6 a.m. and 10 a.m. and 6 p.m. and 10 p.m.

- Use your dry brush (see page 86) and/or perform your oil massage (see page 86).

- Shower or bathe using natural soaps and shampoo. If you performed an oil massage, you can leave a thin sheen of oil on your skin to block environmental toxins when you venture out; you don't have to scrub off all the oil.

- Eat a warm, nourishing breakfast. Remember not to mix fruit with other food, because

To save time and keep your routine flowing, consider keeping an electric kettle in your bathroom to heat water for drinking and other routines. I have an Ayurvedic bench in my bathroom to make my routine easier. What's on my bench? A kettle, apple cider vinegar, coconut oil, abhyanga oil, Ayurvedic herbal powders and tablets, essential oils, a dry brush, a neti pot, nasya oil, measuring spoons, ramekins for mixing powders, a small glass, and baking soda.

fruit digests at a different rate. One good idea is to eat your fruit before or after you meditate. This will give the fruit time to digest (it needs 45 minutes), so your body has more digestive juices ready for your main meal, after you shower.

- Eat the largest meal of the day sometime between 10 a.m. and 2 p.m., Pitta time of day. If your morning routine takes you past 10 a.m., try to make this your most nutrient-dense meal of the day. Think of it as a late breakfast or early lunch. Allow 4 to 5 hours before your next meal. That might mean you eat two meals on some days, and three on others, depending on when you eat breakfast. It's okay to occasionally eat only two meals on some days, especially for Kapha.

Midday

- The best time to perform concentrated work that requires either mental or physical attention is Pitta time, 10 a.m. to 2 p.m.

- Eat lunch mindfully—your largest meal of the day. This is a good time of day to eat protein.

- Walk for 5 or 10 minutes after your meal to promote digestion.

- A great time for creative work is between 2 p.m. and 6 p.m., Vata time of day.

Evening Routine

- A quick rinse or shower before dinner, if necessary, is a nice way to "wash off the day."

- Eat a light meal for dinner, between 5 p.m. and 7 p.m. (Kapha time of day is 6 p.m. to 10 p.m.)

- Walk for 5 or 10 minutes after your meal to promote digestion.

- Perform calming activities, like folding laundry, reading a book, or listening to music.

- Take your triphala (see page 143) and drink Golden Milk (see page 60) before bed.

- Floss and brush your teeth.

- Be in bed by 9 p.m. or 10 p.m. This is also the best time of day for sex (see page 127).

- Journal any thoughts running through your head so they won't disturb your sleep.

- Oil your ears, head, and feet to calm the nervous system and promote deep sleep (see page 86).

- Apply essential oils such as nutmeg or lavender (good for all doshas) to help with sleep (see page 90).

- Practice a calming pranayama with mantras (see page 110) before falling asleep.

- Try to be asleep by 10 p.m. or 11 p.m. (Pitta time of night is 10 p.m. to 2 a.m.)

- If you wake during the night, do some breath work or chant a mantra (see page 110) to help you fall back asleep.

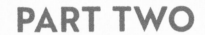

PART TWO

A Wide Range of Ayurvedic Healing Methods

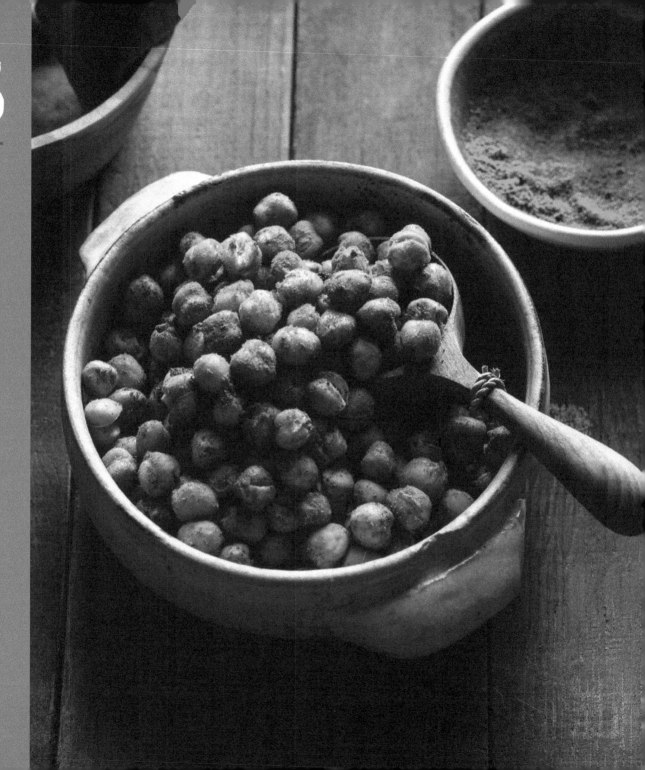

CHAPTER 5

Healing Ayurvedic Recipes

Most of the recipes in this chapter are one-pot meals that are usually complete meals on their own. The combination of oils, spices, beans, grains, and greens creates wholesome, hearty, and nutritionally complete dishes. All of these recipes are vegetarian, but in Ayurveda, we do take into account that some people need meat on occasion. If you are not used to vegetarian dishes, just try these out for a few meals a week.

You will notice that no raw-food recipes are included. In Ayurveda, we prefer food to be at least slightly cooked or steamed, to make the digestive process easier. When we eat raw food, the body uses an enormous amount of energy to break it down and digest it. By cooking our food (and chewing it well), we help our body begin the digestive process. That way, we can immediately use the nutrients and conserve energy for other parts of our body and mind that need healing and restoration. Try eating this way for a few weeks and notice how good you feel.

EVERYDAY CCF TEA

Vata, Pitta & Kapha pacifying

YIELD: **5 servings**   PREP: **3 minutes**   COOK: **5 minutes**

This easy-to-make tea is profoundly healing. The mix of cumin, coriander, and fennel helps kindle your digestive "fire" (agni), improve digestion, nourish the tissues, and keep cravings at bay. At Ayurvedic conferences and lectures, they often serve this tea for attendees to sip all day long.

5 cups water

1 teaspoon cumin seeds

1 teaspoon coriander seeds

1 teaspoon fennel seeds

½ teaspoon ajwain seeds (optional)

1. In a small pot, add the water and seeds. Stir.

2. Bring to a boil, and let it simmer for 5 minutes. Remove from the heat and strain.

3. Pour the tea into a mug, and enjoy.

I often make a pot of tea in the morning, adjusting the amount of seeds to the amount of water I use. I mix the seeds together beforehand in equal amounts and use 1 teaspoon of the seed mixture per cup of water.

GHEE

Vata & Pitta pacifying, Kapha use in moderation

YIELD: about 10 ounces   **COOK:** 15 to 25 minutes (varies)

This magical elixir is the base of so many Ayurvedic recipes, medicines, and healing practices. Ghee is believed to be the only oil that carries the nutrients in food and spices through all seven layers of our tissues: plasma, blood, bones, muscles, fat, nervous system, and reproductive system. Ghee is also a high-heat cooking oil. It activates many healing qualities in spices, which is why spices are sautéed in ghee as one of the first steps in many recipes. Once you master making ghee, you can try it with different spices and herbs, such as clove buds, garlic, or cilantro. Some people find making ghee intimidating, but by staying present, using all your senses, and preparing ghee in a loving, caring way, your ghee will be delicious, nutritious, and healing.

1 pound (4 sticks) of organic, unsalted butter

1. Place the butter in a saucepan, preferably one with a heavy bottom. Turn the heat to medium, and watch the butter as it melts. Ghee requires all of your senses, so do not step away.

2. As the butter begins to melt, lower the heat to medium-low, and stir occasionally, or even not at all. White foam will form on the top as the milk solids separate from the butter, and fine steam will rise as the water evaporates. The butter will begin to sputter, the sounds becoming loud and rapid.

3. Ghee cooking time varies depending on your altitude, the type of butter, and the stove and pot being used, but after about 10 to 15 minutes, you will notice the ghee beginning to quiet down. The color will change to a deep golden hue, and the milk solids will settle at the bottom of the pan and begin to turn brown, and become very aromatic. As soon as the ghee quiets down and only a few bubbles are present, it is done. At this point, remove the pot from the heat. The milk solids burn quickly, so pay attention.

4. Allow the very hot ghee to cool off for a few minutes in the pot.

5. Carefully pour the ghee through a fine mesh sieve into a Pyrex glass or stainless-steel ghee container, if you have one, to cool off even further. Do not pour the ghee directly into a glass jar until it has cooled off significantly, or the jar will crack. If you must pour it into a jar immediately, place a metal spoon in the jar to absorb the heat.

6. The curds at the bottom of the pot can be given to your pet as a treat in small amounts, or you can add a bit of Indian boiled sugarcane solids, called *jaggery,* to them for a delightful treat.

Do not refrigerate ghee, and do not get it wet. Ghee has an incredibly long shelf life when kept covered and dry. Never use a wet knife or spoon to scoop out your ghee, as it will spoil it. Ghee that has been aged 100 years is sold in India as medicine, but yours doesn't need to age to have incredible health benefits.

GOLDEN MILK

Vata, Pitta & Kapha pacifying

YIELD: 1 serving   **PREP:** 2 minutes   **COOK:** 5 minutes

Golden milk is an age-old recipe that nourishes the body on many levels. Turmeric helps reduce inflammation, ghee distributes the healing properties throughout the body, and trypto-phan in the milk will help you sleep. It is calmative, restorative, and delicious. You can make this a vegan drink by substituting milk and ghee with almond oil and a dairy alternative (such as almond milk, hemp milk, or coconut milk made without zinc oxide).

6 to 8 ounces whole-fat goat's milk
(for Kapha and Pitta) or cow's milk (Vata)

½ teaspoon ghee

½ teaspoon turmeric powder

½ teaspoon ginger powder

1 pinch ground black pepper

1 pinch ground cinnamon

1 pinch ground nutmeg (to promote sleep)

1 small piece jaggery (optional)

1. Add all the ingredients to a small pot. Over medium-high heat, bring the mixture to a boil, then lower the heat and simmer for a minute or two.

2. Pour into a mug, and drink before bed. If you want to enjoy this drink during the day, leave out the nutmeg.

TIP: If you are experiencing constipation, adding more ghee to the milk will help you be good to go!

VATA KITCHARI

Vata pacifying

YIELD: 4 servings   **PREP:** 10 minutes (plus soaking time)   **COOK:** 20 to 30 minutes

The first Ayurvedic dish I made was kitchari from Amadea Morningstar's Ayurvedic Cookbook. I bought all the exotic ingredients. I had no idea what I was doing, but I was determined to begin living an Ayurvedic lifestyle. When I sat down to eat it and took my first spoonful, my entire body said "mmmmm." It felt like my gut and brain finally found some-thing that was thoroughly filling on every level—emotionally, spiritually, and physically. I truly felt complete, and I hope you will, too. This recipe is good for seasonal cleanses as well as just calming down the mind and body. It's good to eat for breakfast, lunch, and dinner.

½ cup dried split yellow mung beans (dal)

½ cup uncooked white basmati rice

2 cups chopped vegetables (one or two types, see choices on next page)

2 tablespoons ghee

1 teaspoon black mustard seeds

1 pinch hing

½ teaspoon cumin seeds

½ teaspoon ajwain seeds

½ teaspoon ground coriander

1 teaspoon turmeric powder

1 small yellow onion, chopped

1 clove garlic, chopped

1 (2-inch) piece fresh ginger, peeled, and grated or minced

4 to 6 cups water ⊗

1 teaspoon sea salt ⊗⊗

½ teaspoon pepper

1 additional teaspoon ghee (optional)

1 teaspoon Bragg's Liquid Aminos (optional)

1 small handful chopped fresh cilantro (for garnish)

➤

1. Place the beans and rice in a bowl of water, and rinse until the water runs relatively clear. Fill the bowl with water, and allow the beans and rice to soak while you prepare the recipe, for up to an hour.

2. Wash and chop the vegetables.

3. Before starting the *vagar* (oil-spice mixture), turn on the exhaust fan over the stove, as spices can give off a strong aroma. Then in a 6-quart soup pot over medium-high heat, heat the ghee. Add the black mustard seeds. When they pop, add the hing, cumin seeds, ajwain seeds, coriander, and turmeric. Cook for about 1 minute, or until aromatic. Spices burn quickly; do not allow them to smoke.

4. Stir the onion, garlic, and ginger into the vagar.

5. Drain the rice and beans, and add them to the vagar. Stir until the rice and beans are coated. Allow to sit for 1 to 2 minutes, stirring occasionally.

6. Add the water to the pot, and stir. Add the vegetables, and stir again. Cover the pot, and bring to a boil over medium-high heat.

7. Lower the heat to a simmer. Place the lid askew to let out steam (which lets out excess Vata). Simmer until the water is absorbed, about 15 minutes, or until the kitchari is the consistency you desire.

8. Add the salt and pepper toward the end of cooking.

9. Remove from the heat. Divide into four portions. If using, add more ghee and Bragg's Liquid Aminos to the portion you will eat right away. Then garnish the single portion with cilantro, if using.

⊛ *Use less water for a stew-like consistency or more water for a soupier consistency.*

⊛⊛ *It is important to use sea salt for the extra moisture provided. Do not use Himalayan salt in this recipe.*

Ideal vegetables for this dish include squash, green beans, beets, okra, daikon radish, carrots, peas, and sweet potatoes. To reheat uneaten portions, add some water to the pot and heat over a medium heat. Never microwave or freeze.

PITTA KITCHARI

Pitta pacifying

YIELD: 4 servings   **PREP:** 10 minutes (plus soaking time)   **COOK:** 20 to 30 minutes

Much like the Vata version, in the sense that it's completely nourishing and satisfying, this Pitta-pacifying recipe includes cooling herbs and spices to help balance Pitta on every level. By removing the heating spices like black mustard seeds and hing, and adding in some cooling elements like garnishing with cilantro and coconut, Pitta can enjoy this feel-good comfort food without overheating. Pitta can even allow the dish to cool down a bit before eating.

½ cup dried split yellow mung beans (dal)

½ cup dried white basmati rice

2 cups chopped vegetables (one or two types, see choices on next page)

2 tablespoons ghee

½ teaspoon cumin seeds

½ teaspoon ground coriander

½ teaspoon fennel seeds

1 teaspoon turmeric powder

1 small yellow onion, chopped

1 (1-inch) piece fresh ginger, peeled, and grated or minced

4 to 6 cups water ⊗

1 teaspoon sea salt ⊗ ⊗

1 additional teaspoon ghee (optional)

1 teaspoon Bragg's Liquid Aminos (optional)

1 small handful chopped fresh cilantro (optional)

1 to 2 tablespoons unsweetened shredded coconut (optional)

➤

1. Place the beans and rice in a bowl of water, and rinse until the water runs relatively clear. Fill the bowl with water, and allow the beans and rice to soak while you prepare the recipe, for up to an hour.

2. Wash and chop the vegetables.

3. Before starting the *vagar* (oil-spice mixture), turn on the exhaust fan over the stove, as spices can give off a strong aroma. Then in a 6-quart soup pot over medium-high heat, heat the ghee. Add the cumin, coriander, fennel, and turmeric. Cook for about 1 minute, or until aromatic. Spices burn quickly; do not allow them to smoke.

4. Stir in the onion and ginger. Allow the onion to become tender to sweeten it up for Pitta.

5. Drain the rice and beans, and add them to the vagar. Stir until the rice and beans are coated. Allow to sit for 1 to 2 minutes, stirring occasionally.

6. Add the water to the pot, and stir. Add the vegetables, and stir again. Cover the pot, and bring to a boil over medium-high heat.

7. Lower the heat to a simmer. Simmer until the water is absorbed, about 15 minutes, or until the kitchari is the consistency you desire.

8. Add the salt toward the end of cooking.

9. Remove from the heat. Divide into four portions. If using, add ghee and Bragg's Liquid Aminos to the portion you will eat right away. Garnish the single portion with cilantro and/or coconut, if desired.

⊛ *Use less water for a stew-like consistency or more water for a soupier consistency.*

⊛⊛ *It is important to use sea salt for the extra moisture provided. Do not use Himalayan salt in this recipe.*

Ideal vegetable choices for this dish include burdock root, zucchini, green beans, asparagus, carrots, and celery. To reheat uneaten portions, add some water to the pot and heat over a medium heat. Never microwave or freeze.

KAPHA KITCHARI

Kapha pacifying

YIELD: 4 servings   **PREP:** 10 minutes   **COOK:** 20 to 30 minutes

This extremely nourishing meal can be eaten for breakfast, lunch, and dinner. It is ideal for a mono-fast during a cleanse. In Kapha kitchari, we use less ghee than for the other two doshas, but it is still an important ingredient for a satisfying meal, as the ghee deposits nutrients deep down into all seven layers of your tissues. A little bit of ghee goes a long way! Kapha can also speed up the cooking process by preparing over a higher heat. Just stay present and stir more frequently. The fast cooking time may translate into helping Kapha speed up a bit!

½ cup dried split yellow mung beans (dal)

½ cup dried white basmati rice
or ½ cup uncooked quinoa

2 cups chopped vegetables and/or leafy greens (two or three types, see choices on next page)

3 carrots, chopped

2 celery stalks, chopped

1 teaspoon ghee

1 teaspoon black mustard seeds

½ teaspoon cumin seeds

½ teaspoon ground coriander

½ teaspoon ajwain seeds

½ teaspoon ground cinnamon

½ teaspoon ground cloves, or
2 to 3 whole clove buds

1 pinch hing

1 teaspoon turmeric powder

1 to 2 cloves garlic, chopped

1 (2-inch) piece fresh ginger, peeled and grated or minced

1 small yellow onion, chopped

4 to 6 cups water ⊛

1 to 2 teaspoons Himalayan salt ⊛⊛

1 teaspoon pepper

1 teaspoon Bragg's Liquid Aminos (optional)

1 small handful chopped fresh cilantro (for garnish)

➤

1. Place the beans and rice or quinoa in a bowl of water, and rinse until the water runs relatively clear. Fill the bowl with water, and allow the beans and rice or quinoa to soak while you prepare the recipe, for up to an hour.

2. Wash and chop the vegetables, carrots, and celery.

3. Before starting the *vagar* (oil-spice mixture), turn on the exhaust fan over the stove, as spices can give off a strong aroma. Then in a 6-quart soup pot over medium-high heat, heat the ghee. Add the black mustard seeds. When they pop, add the cumin, coriander, ajwain, cinnamon, cloves, hing, and turmeric. Cook for about 1 minute, or until aromatic. Spices burn quickly; do not allow them to smoke.

4. Stir in the garlic, ginger, and onion.

5. Drain the rice or quinoa and beans, and add them to the vagar. Stir until the rice or quinoa and beans are coated. Allow to sit for 1 to 2 minutes, stirring occasionally.

6. Add the water to the pot, and stir. Add the vegetables, carrots, and celery, and stir again. Cover the pot, and bring to a boil over medium-high heat. (If using leafy greens, add them in step 7.)

7. Lower the heat to a simmer. Simmer until the water is absorbed, about 15 minutes, or until the kitchari is the consistency you desire. Just before removing the pot from the heat, add the greens and stir until wilted.

8. Add the salt and pepper toward the end of cooking.

9. Remove from the heat. Divide into four portions. If using, add Bragg's Liquid Aminos to the portion you will eat right away. Garnish the single portion with cilantro, if desired.

⊗ *Use less water for a stew-like consistency or more water for a soupier consistency.*

⊗⊗ *It is important to use Himalayan salt in this recipe; sea salt will add more water to already watery Kapha, which is undesired.*

Ideal vegetable choices for this dish include burdock root, cauliflower, broccoli, white potato, daikon radish, green beans, spinach, kale, mustard greens, and chard. To reheat uneaten portions, add some water to the pot and heat over a medium heat. Never microwave or freeze.

How to Eat Warm Kitchari at Work

How do you eat a hearty warm lunch at the office? Instead of using the microwave, which destroys the nutrients in food, buy a Thermos. Heat your food up on the stove in the morning, put it in the Thermos, and leave it on your desk until lunchtime. Your food will be piping hot. You can also use an Indian Tiffin. This stackable container unit is ubiquitous in India. Made of stainless steel, three, four, five or more compartments can be stacked on top of each other. Typically one contains rice, dal, chapatti (unleavened flat bread), vegetables, and maybe a sweet. To help keep the food warm, wrap the tiffin in a towel before packing it in your bag. It won't keep your food as hot as a Thermos will, but the food won't get too cold, either.

BOK CHOY, TEMPEH, AND MUSHROOM STIR-FRY

Vata & Pitta nourishing, Kapha increasing

YIELD: 4 servings   PREP: 10 minutes   COOK: 20 minutes

Bok choy is also known as Chinese cabbage. Part of the cruciferous vegetable family, it packs a nutritious punch of antioxidants and vitamin A, which can help reduce stress in the body and promote cancer prevention. I love the subtle crunch and fresh flavor it adds to any dish. Combining bok choy with mushrooms and tempeh creates a variety of textures in the mouth— even though each flavor is mild, they are supportive of the others. Kapha can enjoy bok choy in a variety of ways, including sautéing, in soup, and even chopped raw in a summer salad.

1 tablespoon sesame seed oil

3 tablespoons toasted sesame oil, divided

½ onion, chopped

2 celery stalks, chopped

2 carrots, chopped

1 (1-inch) piece fresh ginger, cut into matchsticks

1 small jalapeño, veined, seeded, and chopped (omit for Pitta)

½ cup dried organic shitake mushrooms, presoaked for 30 minutes

½ cup chopped organic portobello mushroom, or mushroom of choice

1 tablespoon sesame seeds

3 tablespoons tamari sauce, divided

2 baby bok choy heads

1 (8-ounce) package of tempeh, cubed

1. In a large skillet over medium heat, heat the sesame seed oil and 1 tablespoon of the toasted sesame seed oil.

2. Add the onion and sauté until it is translucent, about 2 to 3 minutes.

3. Add the celery, carrots, ginger, jalapeño, shitake mushrooms, and portobello mushroom or your mushroom of choice. Cook for 5 minutes, stirring occasionally.

4. Sprinkle the sesame seeds on top, and add 1 tablespoon of the tamari sauce. Lay the bok choy over the mixture and let sit for 1 minute before stirring in.

5. Cover the pan, and let sit for another 5 minutes, or until the bok choy is soft.

6. In a separate pan, sauté the tempeh with the remaining toasted sesame oil and tamari sauce. Cook for 5 minutes, or until the tempeh is lightly browned.

7. Mix together the vegetables and tempeh mixture, and divide into four servings.

KAPHA TIP: Tempeh is considered a heavy food, but it is also drying and astringent, so it can have benefits for Vata, Pitta, and Kapha; however, Kapha should use it in moderation. Kapha should use ½ tablespoon of sesame oil, 1½ tablespoons of toasted sesame oil, and half of a package of tempeh in place of the amounts listed.

INGREDIENT TIP: Mushrooms should *always* be cooked. Uncooked mushrooms are indigestible and can create toxins in the body. Since mushrooms absorb the minerals and nutrients in the soil, they can also absorb toxins. Always buy organic.

DAIKON AND TOFU SUMMER DETOX SOUP

Vata, Pitta & Kapha pacifying (with dosha-specific ingredients)

YIELD: 4 servings   **PREP:** 15 minutes   **COOK:** 10 to 15 minutes

This is a great summertime soup, as the fennel and cumin are cooling. The benefits of mild daikon radish include healthy digestion, and it may also help improve blood circulation and prevent clots. The juice extracted from raw daikon has been traditionally used to alleviate headaches, fever, swollen gums, and hot flashes. It has anti-inflammatory and cooling effects. Daikon radish also contains high amounts of potassium, vitamin C, and phosphorus—nutrients that are essential for good health. Even in the summer, warm soup can feel so satisfying. Eat this soup for breakfast to begin your day with a warm feeling in your tummy that will last well into lunchtime.

1 tablespoon olive oil or ghee

1 teaspoon toasted sesame seed oil

½ onion, chopped

1 cup chopped mushrooms of choice

1 (5-inch) piece fresh daikon radish, sliced and halved

1 cup black or kidney beans, or ½ cup red lentils (for Kapha), or 8 ounces firm tofu, cubed (for Vata and Pitta)

1 teaspoon minced fresh ginger

2 cloves garlic, minced (for Vata and Kapha), or 1 clove garlic, minced (for Pitta)

½ teaspoon turmeric powder

½ teaspoon ajwain seeds

1 teaspoon fennel seeds

1 teaspoon cumin seeds

2 cups vegetable broth

1 cup organic miso broth

1 cup water

Dash Himalayan salt (for Kapha) or sea salt (for Vata and Pitta)

Freshly ground black pepper, to taste

Sprigs of cilantro for garnish (optional)

1. In a 6-quart soup pot, add the olive oil or ghee and toasted sesame seed oil. Heat over medium-low heat.

2. Add the onion, mushrooms, daikon radish, beans (or lentils or tofu), ginger, and garlic. Sauté until aromatic and the vegetables are softened.

3. Mix in the turmeric, ajwain, fennel, and cumin. Add the vegetable broth, miso broth, and water, and bring to a boil over medium-high heat.

4. Turn the heat down, and simmer for about 10 minutes.

5. Add the salt and pepper. Divide into four servings, and garnish with cilantro, if desired.

Serve over half a cup of cooked white basmati or jasmine rice, if you'd like. You may even want to top with some raw or home-roasted pumpkin seeds.

WINTER-WARMING WHOLE MUNG BEAN SOUP

Vata, Pitta & Kapha nourishing

YIELD: 4 servings   **PREP:** 15 minutes (plus soaking time overnight)   **COOK:** 60 minutes

There is something indescribably satisfying about mung beans, so it is no wonder that many cultures call them their own. Whole mung beans are green, unlike the split version, which are yellow. Mung, which packs a nutritious punch, is called the "mighty mung bean" for good reason: The little green bean and its yellow counterpart contain a host of minerals, including folate, manganese, magnesium, iron, thiamine, copper, zinc, and potassium. It also includes vitamins A, C, B_6, B_{12}, E, and K. How can they not be delicious? When the body recognizes how good a food is for it, it embraces the food. That's how I feel about mung. I'm crazy about it!

1 cup dried green whole mung beans

6 to 8 cups water (depending on desired consistency)

1 strip kombu

2 tablespoons olive oil, or avocado oil or ghee

½ teaspoon black mustard seeds

1 teaspoon cumin seeds

1 teaspoon ajwain seeds, or celery seeds

1 teaspoon ground cumin

1 teaspoon turmeric powder

4 to 6 fresh or frozen curry leaves (optional)

1 small yellow onion, chopped

2 to 3 garlic cloves, chopped (for Vata and Kapha), or 2 garlic cloves chopped (for Pitta)

1 tablespoon roughly chopped fresh ginger

1 to 2 cups organic vegetable broth (optional)

2 carrots, chopped

2 celery stalks, chopped

1 to 2 yellow potatoes, cubed

1 small green jalapeño, deveined, seeds removed, and chopped

½ lemon

Fresh parsley or cilantro, chopped, for garnish (optional)

1 teaspoon ghee (optional for Vata and Pitta, less for Kapha)

1. Soak the mung beans in water overnight.

2. Rinse the beans and place them in a 6-quart pot. Add the water and kombu. Bring to a boil over medium-high heat. This will take about 45 minutes. Discard the kombu, and set the pot aside.

3. In a small sauce pan, add the olive oil, or avocado oil or ghee. Heat the pan to medium heat.

4. Add the black mustard seeds. When the mustard seeds pop, add the cumin seeds, ajwain, cumin powder, turmeric, and curry leaves, if using. Stir quickly.

5. Add the onion, garlic, and ginger. Over medium heat, being careful not to let anything burn, cook for about 5 to 10 minutes, or until the onion becomes translucent. Then add the mixture to the pot of beans.

6. Add a few more cups of water or organic vegetable broth, if desired, to increase the liquid content. Add the carrots, celery, potatoes, and jalapeño. Bring to a boil over medium-high heat, and then lower to a simmer. Simmer for about 15 minutes, and remove from the heat.

7. Use an immersion blender to roughly blend the soup, or transfer in small batches to a countertop blender, being careful to allow steam to escape between pulses. Just a few pulses will do.

8. Before serving, squeeze in the juice of half a lemon. Garnish with chopped parsley or cilantro, if desired, and a teaspoon of ghee (less for Kapha), if using, before serving.

URAD DAL PORRIDGE

Vata pacifying; Vata, Pitta & Kapha benefit after travel

YIELD: 4 servings   **PREP:** 10 minutes   **COOK:** 30 minutes

Urad dal, also known as black gram, is a heavy type of dal that is great for calming Vata. This recipe is perfect to make after traveling—whether it's a 13-hour trip to India or a 5-hour coast-to-coast flight—all travelers can benefit from the grounding, heating qualities of urad dal. As airplane travel dries you out, urad dal counteracts that with its moist, unctuous, heating qualities. While those qualities tend to increase Pitta and Kapha, I find that using this recipe just after travel can benefit all doshas. Vata can also add another spoonful of ghee before eating.

1 cup uncooked white basmati rice

1 cup dried split urad dal

2 tablespoons white, brown, or red miso paste

3 cups vegetable broth, mushroom broth, or a combination

1 to 2 cups water (depending on desired consistency)

1 tablespoon ghee

½ medium yellow onion, chopped

1 teaspoon garlic powder

1 teaspoon turmeric powder

½ teaspoon ground cumin

½ teaspoon ground coriander

4 to 5 leaves Swiss chard, rainbow chard, kale, or mustard greens, chopped

½ teaspoon sea salt

Freshly ground black or white pepper

½ teaspoon Bragg's Liquid Aminos (optional)

2 tablespoons raw, unsalted pumpkin seeds, or sunflower seeds, for garnish (optional)

1. In a bowl, mix the rice and dal together and rinse well. Fill the bowl with water and allow the dal and rice to soak while you prepare the other ingredients.

2. Boil ½ cup of hot water, pour into a small bowl, and stir in the miso paste until it dissolves.

3. In an 8-quart soup pot, add the miso broth, vegetable broth, and water, and heat over medium heat.

4. Add the ghee, onion, garlic powder, turmeric, cumin, and coriander to the broth.

5. Bring to a boil, and add the soaked rice and dal. Allow the mixture to come to a boil again, and then lower to a simmer and cover the pot. Stir occasionally until all the liquid is absorbed.

6. Toward the end of cooking, add the greens and stir well. Cover the pot and allow the greens to wilt over very low heat or no heat.

7. Add the salt and pepper. Let the porridge sit for about 5 minutes. Divide into four servings and, if desired, top each serving with the Bragg's Liquid Aminos and the pumpkin or sunflower seeds.

To make this recipe vegan, use avocado oil instead of ghee. Refrigerate remaining portions and reconstitute it by adding more water or broth the next day before reheating over medium heat.

EASY BREAKFAST BOWL

Vata, Pitta & Kapha pacifying (with dosha-specific ingredients)

YIELD: 2 servings   **PREP:** 5 minutes   **COOK:** 15 minutes

One of the most popular questions I hear is, "What should I eat for breakfast?" Since Ayurveda doesn't like mixing fruit with other foods, because they digest at different rates, people can be confused over things like yogurt with fruit, oatmeal with berries, or cold cereal with sliced fruit. So here is a recommendation: Eat your fruit about 45 minutes before your main meal so that it does not disturb your digestion. Try this porridge anytime of year. It's deeply satisfying and should give you long-lasting energy throughout the morning.

1 cup quinoa (for Pitta or Kapha), or 1 cup millet (for Kapha), or 1 cup rice (for Vata)

2 cups water

½ cup goat's milk (for Pitta, Kapha, and Vata), or almond milk (for Vata)

1 teaspoon ground cinnamon

¼ teaspoon ground nutmeg

¼ teaspoon ginger powder

½ teaspoon pea protein powder, chia seeds, or ground flaxseeds (optional for power boost)

1 tablespoon maple syrup or honey

1 teaspoon ghee (optional for Vata and Pitta) or ½ teaspoon ghee (optional for Kapha)

1. Rinse the quinoa, millet, or rice well. In a 4-quart sauce pan, combine the grain and water, and bring to a boil over medium heat. Lower the heat to a simmer and cover. Simmer until all the water is absorbed.

2. In a separate 2-quart saucepan, add the milk, cinnamon, nutmeg, and ginger, and heat gently over low heat.

3. Divide the grain into two servings, and pour an even amount of the hot milk and spices on top.

4. If using the optional power boost, stir half the pea protein powder, chia seeds, or flaxseeds into each bowl.

5. Add the maple syrup or honey and the ghee, if using.

Either stick with the grain or seed recommended for your dosha or choose your grain or seed seasonally. In the winter, use millet or rice, and in the spring and summer, use quinoa.

CHICKPEA PICK-ME-UP

Vata, Pitta & Kapha pacifying

YIELD: 4 servings   **PREP:** 15 minutes (plus soaking time)   **COOK:** 45 to 60 minutes

Chickpeas, also known as garbanzo beans, are one of the most versatile beans. Their light, dry quality makes them a perfect choice for Pitta and Kapha, but not such a great choice for Vata. This little legume contains fiber, protein, manganese, folate, copper, phosphorus, iron, and even a bit of zinc, making it an extremely healthy choice that is also low in calories and fat. They are also easy to cook with. Their slightly nutty, sweet flavor is delicious and subtle, allowing the chickpea to absorb the spices it is cooked with.

1 cup dried organic chickpeas

4 cups water (for soaking)

1 piece kombu

3 cups water (for cooking)

1 to 2 tablespoons sunflower oil

1 teaspoon black mustard seeds

1 pinch hing

1 teaspoon turmeric powder

1 teaspoon cumin seeds

1 teaspoon fennel seeds

½ teaspoon ground cumin

½ teaspoon ground coriander

1 small yellow onion, chopped

2 cloves garlic, minced

4 curry leaves (optional)

1 cup chopped tomatoes (optional for Vata, omit for Pitta and Kapha)

6 to 8 kale leaves

Himalayan salt

Freshly ground black pepper

➤

1. Add the dried chickpeas to the water with the kombu, and soak overnight, or for at least 8 hours.

2. Drain and rinse the chickpeas, reserving the kombu. Add the chickpeas, kombu, and water to a 6-quart pot. Cover the pot, and bring to a boil over medium-high heat. Reduce to a simmer, and cook until the chickpeas are tender, about 30 to 45 minutes.

3. Drain the chickpeas, reserving ½ cup of the water, and discard the kombu.

4. In a large frying pan, heat the oil over medium heat. Add the black mustard seeds. Once they pop, add the hing, turmeric, cumin seeds, fennel, ground cumin, and coriander. Stir quickly.

5. Add the onion, and cook for about 5 minutes, or until tender.

6. Stir in the garlic and the curry leaves (if using).

7. Add the chickpeas to the pan, and stir until well coated.

8. Add the reserved cooking water if preferred, for a soupier consistency, or leave it out.

9. Add the tomatoes, if using.

10. Layer the kale leaves over the mix and allow to wilt, about 5 minutes. Cover the pan and let the spices and flavors meld for about 5 to 8 minutes, stirring occasionally.

11. Add the salt and pepper. Serve.

If Pitta and Kapha want to enjoy this dish even more, add a big handful of fresh cilantro before serving. Vata can use more oil when cooking or add some ghee before eating.

Always use non-GMO organic chickpeas, as the nonorganic type has loads of pesticides applied. You can use 1 (8-ounce) can of chickpeas in place of the dried chickpeas. Be sure to purchase only BPA-free, non-GMO, organic, canned chickpeas and rinse them well before using.

CRUNCHY CHICKPEAS

Pitta & Kapha pacifying

YIELD: 5 cups   **PREP:** 20 minutes   Cooking: 30 minutes

While we don't promote snacking in Ayurveda, sometimes we just need a little something to peck on now and then. Crunchy garbanzo beans make a satisfying and supremely healthy choice for Pitta and Kapha. As witnessed by the many packaged chickpea snacks now commonly seen in stores, chickpeas are popular these days. You can make this snack yourself for a quarter of the price. You can also customize the flavors to satisfy your dosha, and your palate, by getting creative with the spices.

2 cups precooked chickpeas, or 2 (8-ounce) cans chickpeas, drained and rinsed

1 teaspoon sea salt (for Pitta), or Himalayan salt (for Kapha)

½ teaspoon smoked paprika, or ½ teaspoon ground cumin, or ½ teaspoon garam masala powder (optional)

1 tablespoon sunflower or safflower oil (optional for crunchiness; no oil for Kapha)

1. Spread the rinsed chickpeas on a baking sheet to dry, about 20 minutes.

2. Preheat the oven to 450°F.

3. In a mixing bowl, add the chickpeas; salt; paprika, cumin, or garam masala (if using); and the oil (if using). Toss well to coat, and spread on a baking sheet in a single layer.

4. Place the baking sheet in the oven and bake for 20 minutes. Remove from the oven, and use a spatula to turn the chickpeas over. Place back in the oven and roast for an additional 10 minutes, or until the chickpeas are slightly browned. Roast a little longer, if desired, for crunchier chickpeas.

Store the crunchy chickpeas in an airtight container. Do not refrigerate. These are great to sprinkle on salads and rice dishes. Don't make more than you can eat in three days.

To cook your Crunchy Chickpeas, soak overnight, drain, and place into a large soup pot. Cover with water, at least double the amount of beans. Bring to a boil, then cover and simmer for at least 30 to 45 minutes. Check on the beans during cooking. When they are soft, they are done.

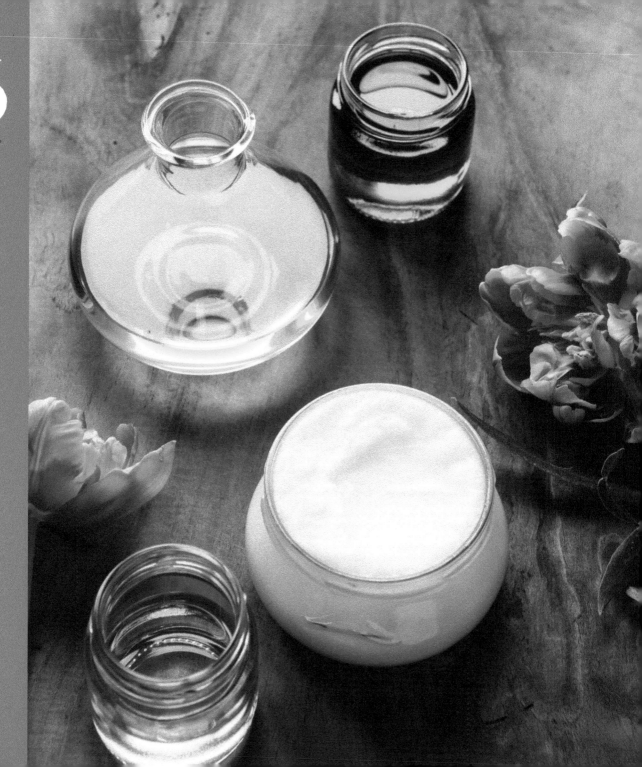

CHAPTER 6

Lifestyle Practices and Yoga Poses

This chapter introduces you to eight lifestyle practices, some of which you may choose to include in your daily routine. Many take only a few minutes to perform, but make such a difference for the rest of the day. Once you start incorporating these practices on a trial basis, you may discover that you don't want to give them up, because they feel so good. What else feels good and carries many health benefits? Yoga. So in this chapter, you will also find several yoga poses (*asanas*) with step-by-step instructions, along with some dosha-specific tips.

TONGUE SCRAPING

First thing in the morning, before taking liquid or food, stick your tongue way out and look in the mirror. If your tongue has a white (Kapha), yellowish (Pitta), or blackish (Vata) coating, you have some toxins in your digestive system. This coating is a great way to get an indication of which dosha might be out of balance. But if your tongue looks pink and clear—you are doing great! Nevertheless, a tongue scraping is still beneficial.

Using a metal tongue scraper, or if you don't have one, the edge of a spoon, scrape your tongue as far back as you can, using gentle pressure, at least seven times, rinsing the scraper between scrapes. Brush your teeth when you're done.

When you scrape your tongue, not only are you removing many toxins and bacteria you accumulated in your mouth overnight, you are actually massaging the organs in the digestive tract, which are represented on each quadrant of the tongue based on Ayurvedic knowledge.

OIL PULLING (GANDUSHA)

Oil pulling is an ancient Ayurvedic technique for cleansing the mouth and body by holding oil in the mouth for 10 to 20 minutes every day, if possible. This is gaining widespread popularity, which is well-deserved. The benefits of oil pulling include reducing "bad" bacteria in the mouth, gums, cheeks, and tongue; preventing bad breath and tooth decay; teeth whitening; and may even help detoxify the entire body. Some say that the oil pulls toxins from the entire body through this procedure, noting that the tongue is connected to all the major organs and other body parts.

In India, it's not unusual to meet people who have never owned a toothbrush yet they have marvelous pearly whites and no cavities. An Indian tradition of teeth brushing is chewing on a stick from the neem tree and oil pulling with coconut oil (in the south) or sesame seed oil (in the north). Both oils have antibacterial properties that help reduce plaque and remove impurities from the mouth.

You can make oil pulling a part of your morning routine. Just keep a jar of organic, unrefined coconut oil (no preservatives) in your bathroom, along with a tablespoon. It's best to perform this task during your morning routine before eating and drinking, as the body has worked hard all night to rid itself of bad bacteria and many of those end up on your tongue and in your cheek tissues.

After scraping your tongue, place a tablespoon of coconut oil in your mouth. It may feel strange at first, but the oil will melt and the real work will begin. As you allow the oil to sit in your mouth, only swishing gently now and then, the lauric acid and other compounds in the oil begin an intense cleansing process. Allow the oil to stay in your mouth for about 10 to 20 minutes. (You may not have time for this every morning, but do try to fit it in when you can.)

When you are done, spit the used oil into a trash can (not in the sink, as you don't want oil to clog your drain). It will have a milky, foamy consistency now. For extra freshness, mix ¼ teaspoon of baking soda with a little water, and do a quick rinse. You will feel sparkling and clean.

DRINK HOT WATER WITH LEMON OR LIME

After cleaning your mouth with a tongue scraper and brushing, drink hot or warm water with a squeeze of lemon (for Kapha and Vata) or lime (for Pitta) in the morning. Waiting until after cleaning your mouth ensures that you won't swallow the bacteria that built up in your mouth overnight.

For Kapha, add 1 teaspoon of raw, organic honey to warm (but not hot) water. Honey is heating and can scrape away excess Kapha. Do not include honey for Pitta and Vata, though. It's too hot for Pitta and too drying for Vata. (On the topic of honey, be sure not to mix honey with hot water and don't cook with it, as it can create ama at high temperatures.)

The hot or warm water hydrates your tissues more effectively than cold water. Lemon acts to alkaline the body. We typically wake up with a high acidic pH level, and lemon, oddly enough, balances that out. Lemon juice also contains potassium, vitamins B and C, calcium, magnesium, and trace minerals. It cleanses the liver and stimulates your digestive fires—and Ayurveda loves that—so you will be ready for a good breakfast or early meal. It will also facilitate a good bowel movement. The water hydrates your tissues after a night of drying out, and also signals the body it's time to "go."

Lime has a more cooling effect, while lemon has a more heating effect. Lime has less acid and is less sour than lemon, so it's a better choice for Pitta, especially. Kapha does well with less sour as well, so lime is a good choice if it's preferred. Limes have slightly more vitamin A than lemons, and a little less vitamin C, but other than that, it is really the acid/sour taste that comes into play with the doshas.

TIP: Cut up a lemon or lime into slices at the beginning of the week, and keep them in an airtight container in the refrigerator, so you aren't tempted to skip it.

A couple of times a week, you may want to use 1 teaspoon of apple cider vinegar in place of the citrus in your warm water. This pleasant-tasting probiotic-fermented elixir is said to be helpful in reducing blood sugar levels, lowering cholesterol, supporting weight loss by improving metabolism, and reducing acid in the system. If the taste is too unpleasant for you, you can stir in a teaspoon of raw honey to sweeten it up.

DRY BRUSHING

A dry brush is typically a natural-bristle brush with a handle for use on the body. Dry brush before you do your oil massage (see page 86) and before you shower. Using a dry brush increases circulation, moves toxins out of the body, and exfoliates the skin.

Begin with your feet, moving the brush upward, using firm pressure. Move in straight lines over the long bones and in circular motions around the joints. Spend more time in areas like the thighs and buttocks, which tend to contain more fat and therefore accumulate more toxins. As you move up your body, reaching your arms and neck, continue brushing upward. Do not use the brush on your face. This should be about a five-minute process.

OIL MASSAGE (ABHYANGA)

Oil massage, or *abhyanga*, is a full-body oil self-massage, which helps stimulate the lymph system and remove toxins. By leaving the oil on the skin for 20 minutes, the oil penetrates all 7 layers of the tissues, helping to remove toxins that are held down deep in the system. There are dosha-specific oils that are infused with herbs to pacify imbalances. (Ready-made dosha-specific blends from several companies are available; see the resources on page 161.) Use only organic oils on your body. This practice is recommended for every dosha, but it can depend on the climate and season. It's best to avoid this practice if you are menstruating, are pregnant, are going through an illness, or have open sores, or infected, swollen skin.

Vata: heavy, heating oils—sesame seed, almond, or avocado

Pitta: light, cooling oils—coconut, olive, sunflower, or ghee

Kapha: invigorating, heating oils—mustard or safflower

To perform abhyanga, follow these instructions:

1. Warm a small bottle of oil (capped tightly) under hot water or place it in a mug of hot water. (You will be using less than a quarter cup to a third cup of oil for the entire process.) Remove your clothing and place a towel or mat on the floor, in case the oil drips.

2. Place some of the oil in your palms and rub them together. Add more oil to your palms as necessary. Apply the oil starting with your scalp, and moving to the soles of your feet. Cover your body with oil, using more oil for Vata than for Kapha. Gently massage the oil into your scalp, face, neck, torso, arms, under-arms, breasts, sides, hips, buttocks, back, thighs, knees, calves, ankles, toes, and the soles of your feet.

3. After you have covered your body with oil, massage your scalp for a minute, use circular motions on your face, rub up and down on all the long bones, and in circular motions around the joints. Be gentle on the breasts. Rub the oil on your belly in a clockwise motion. While you are doing this, send love and healing thoughts to your body, perhaps concentrating on what you perceive as trouble spots. Send those areas extra love!

4. If possible, allow the oil to stay on your skin, from start to finish, for about 10 to 15 minutes. If that is not possible, it's okay.

5. When you finish the massage, wipe your feet on the towel and step into the shower or bath. You will want to rinse off the oil so it carries toxins away with it. You don't need to use soap (except for your high-traffic areas), so you can leave this sheen of oil on your skin to protect you from environmental toxins. We do so much scrubbing of the skin that it removes a lot of our natural oils, so we have to apply moisturizer to replenish the skin. If we let the body do its thing, it will function better.

If you don't have time for a full-body mas-sage, at least do your joints, head, and feet.

NETI POT

A neti pot is a container resembling a small teapot that is used to irrigate and flush out your nasal passages. Your nose is your first line of defense against environmental toxins. A neti pot clears out anything that's blocking your nose hair from protecting you against toxins. Having a neti pot handy is a good idea if you live in a humid climate, have seasonal allergies, or are doing a cleanse. The salt water that's used helps reduce inflammation or irritation in your sinuses, and can wash out allergens. If you live in a dry climate or at high altitude, using a neti pot is not recommended.

When using a neti pot, boil water but allow it to cool down until it's just warm. Add ¼ teaspoon neti salt to your neti pot (salt formulated specifically for this technique, which you can find online and in many stores).

Fill up your neti pot with water, and position your head so that it is tilted toward one shoulder, and your chin is not too far forward or too far back. Breathe through your mouth. Gently pour one potful of water through one of your nostrils. If you feel it in your ear, your head is too far back. If you feel it in your sinuses, your head is too far forward. Breathe naturally though your mouth.

After allowing the water to flow through your nostril, gently blow your nose. Repeat with a full pot on the opposite side. After your final blow, you may want to hang your head forward and do "windmills" with your arms. Or fold forward, grab your left ankle with your right hand and look up to the left. Do the same on the other side.

NASYA OIL

Nasya oil is an herbal-infused oil for use in your nostrils. This can feel good no matter what climate you live in, but it is especially useful if you live in a dry climate. If you don't have nasya oil, you can use organic sesame seed oil (but *not* toasted sesame seed oil) or ghee. Oils made specifically for the nose include Banyan Botanicals brand and Super Nasya from the Ayurvedic Institute as well as SVAyurveda Tridoshic Nasya Oil by Chandi, LLC (see resources on page 161).

To use nasya oil, tilt your head back or lay down and place three to five drops directly into each nostril using a dropper and sniff the oil back. Alternatively, insert a clean pinky and massage the oil into your nasal passages. Pinch and release your nostrils and inhale though the nose and release several times. Massage the nasal passages along your nose and cheeks.

You can do this two to three times a day or as needed. When the nasal passages are cared for this way, it helps block environmental toxins and reduce inflammation. Nasya oil is a must-use on airplanes and in hotel rooms to keep the sinuses moist and healthy. It also feels good to massage the outer nose with the oil. I love to use the extra oil on my finger to massage into my cuticles. My husband uses this oil on his elbows and swears they have never been softer.

IMPORTANT NOTE: Do not use nasya oil until at least an hour after you have used your neti pot so that you don't trap any water in your nasal passages or sinuses.

AROMATHERAPY

Aromatherapy, the therapeutic use of essential oils, is healing and balancing to both the body and the mind. When used on the skin or by inhaling, essential oil infuses the body with tiny molecules that can enter the bloodstream to nourish and heal, calming the nervous system and thereby stimulating the body's natural defenses and inner pharmacy. It's a super practice to learn about and incorporate into your life, not to mention most oils smell good. Keep in mind, though, that using essential oils properly and learning to make blends is a serious process. Make sure to study with a professional before trying to heal yourself of any complicated ailment with essential oils.

Many essential oils have volatile compounds in a concentrated form that can offer therapeutic-level healing in just a few drops. Less is better when working with oils; just a few drops can be highly beneficial. Many essential oils are antimicrobial and antifungal (e.g., tea tree, lavender, and oregano). Some essential oils can repel insects, too (a mix of citronella, lemongrass, and geranium works well). Tea tree and lavender oils are always with me when I travel. If there is room in my luggage, I also take peppermint, ginger, and sandalwood—all of which physically and mentally ease any travel disturbances I encounter, from nausea to fatigue.

Mentally, the sense of smell can invoke memories—both good and bad. Different areas of your brain can be stimulated to heal, release tension, or increase joy depending on the scent you choose. The use of essential oils to evoke these sensory feelings is an Ayurvedic method to create a healing pathway to the brain through the body.

Choosing Your Oils

Essential oils are completely different from fragrance and scented oils, which have zero therapeutic effect and can cause allergies. Choose only 100 percent pure essential oils—look for therapeutic-grade oils, organic oils, or pure plant oils. High-quality oils are becoming more easily available and at better prices. There are several multilevel marketing companies that sell expensive essential oils, but in my experience, you can get a good high-quality oil at your local health food store. Do your research before you buy any essential oils to make sure you are buying high-grade products. Also, be aware that some oils are endangered due to over-harvestation of the plants, including rosewood, sandalwood, and frankincense.

Choose a quality carrier oil to dilute the essential oil if you are using it on your body, as essential oils are quite powerful. (Some undiluted essential oils can be used directly on this skin, but do this only under the advice of a certified aromatherapist.) Using a dosha-specific carrier oil, a list of which follows, will enhance the medicinal qualities of the essential oil and will also make them safer to use.

A good gauge to determine if an oil is right for you is the smile test. Do you smile when you sniff it? If so, use it! Nevertheless, certain oils are best for each dosha. Listed here are single essential oils, but with some knowledge you can create your own blends or purchase ready-made blends for each dosha from places like Floracopeia (see the resources on page 161).

For Vata, choose oils that are warming, grounding, earthy, and sweet, such as vanilla, rose, clove, orange, bergamot, basil, geranium, patchouli, vetiver, fir needle, tangerine, and ylang ylang. The best Vata carrier oils are sesame, avocado, and castor.

For Pitta, choose oils that are sweet, cooling, and calming, such as rose, sandalwood, jasmine, fennel, spearmint, lemon, lavender, lime, lemongrass, tea tree, and neroli. The best Pitta carrier oils are coconut, sunflower, and safflower.

For Kapha, choose invigorating, warming, uplifting, and spicy, such as clove, eucalyptus, rosemary, cinnamon, peppermint, wintergreen, grapefruit, ginger, lemon, lime, and rose. The best Kapha carrier oils are mustard seed (ensure good quality), jojoba, and grapeseed.

Using Your Oils

Use your essential oils or blends in any of the following ways:

- In a diffuser. Diffusing oils in your workspace or at home can quickly change the atmosphere.

- Combine a few drops with a carrier oil or unscented body lotion. Rub on your body as you would any lotion.

- Place a few drops on a cotton ball and inhale deeply a few times.

- Add 10 to 15 drops to your bath.

- Sprinkle a few drops of oil on the walls of your shower before stepping in.

- Fill a bowl with hot water and add a few drops of essential oil. Inhale the steam for a few minutes.

- Make a sweet (Pitta), grounding (Vata), or enlivening (Kapha) spray by adding a few drops of essential oils to a spray bottle filled with distilled water. Spritz your head, neck, and face as needed.

YOGA

Mindful movement can be very fulfilling, because it exercises your brain as much as your body. By staying focused during exercise, we are incorporating the healing process deep into our bones and tissues, and we learn more about what our body wants and when it needs it. I find that yoga—especially Iyengar-style yoga created by BKS Iyengar (1918–2014)—fits the bill for all three doshas.

This particular type of yoga concentrates on alignment, breathing, and proper posture, and is very close to the original practice from centuries ago. Do not confuse yoga postures with yoga from the Vedas. *The Yoga Sutras of Patanjali* is a scripture on living. Yoga *asanas* (postures or poses) are what most of us are familiar with today—putting on yoga attire, grabbing a mat, and heading to a yoga studio.

Almost every pose in yoga can be modified for your particular dosha, and there are certain styles of yoga that are more suited to each type. With that in mind, in the sections that follow, you will find a description of some poses and how they benefit your dosha. (Great thanks go to Dr. David Frawley, author of *Yoga for Your Type: An Ayurvedic Approach to Your Asana Practice*, as well as to Claire Diab, who led my yoga training through the Perfect Health Certification Program at the Chopra Center.)

You will benefit by personalizing your yoga routine to match your primary dosha. A great daily routine will include standing poses, twists, bends, balance, and restorative poses. In addition to yoga, a full workout includes stretching, aerobics, and weight training. (See page 38 for the best forms of exercise for each dosha.)

Vata Yoga Guidelines

Vata, I know you want to fly and flow through your routine, but it's best to slow it down. Those with an overabundance of Vata will greatly benefit from poses that promote grounding, rootedness, and deep breathing. Those poses include Tree Pose, Mountain Pose, and Child's Pose. Warrior 1 and Warrior 2, when held for at least a minute, are also good choices. Each of these poses is described in the next section.

Avoid flow-types of yoga, where you move quickly from one pose to another, which can create anxiety and nervousness in the Vata mind. Vata needs to stay aware of the body in each pose as well as the transitions between poses. Move slowly and deliberately. Avoid the urge to move fast. Forward bends massage the colon and bowel, reducing gas and bloating and promoting healthy elimination—all key to a healthy Vata. "Slow and steady" is the mantra for Vata in yoga.

Vata benefits the most from yoga when they are able to focus and be calm and grounded. Breathe deeply and steadily. Keep it slow and rooted and relaxed. Avoid the urge to flow and move fast. Stay consistent and steady throughout the session. Enjoy a long, deep Corpse Pose at the end of your routine. Since Vata is dry and cold, cover up with a blanket and put on some socks for this pose. Allow the synovial fluid that you got moving in your practice to penetrate deeply into your body.

Pitta Yoga Guidelines

I know you really love hot yoga, but, please, for yourself and all those around you, avoid it! While it might feel good to you initially, you are igniting your Pitta flames, which will throw you off balance in the long run. Rather, choose a yoga routine that is relaxed and cool. Avoid pushing yourself too hard. Choose a studio with no mirrors or music, so you can focus on yourself and not compare yourself to other people. Go within. Be patient and lighthearted with yourself. Enjoy; it's not a competition. Avoid judging yourself or others. With your naturally strong, medium build, yoga poses can be challenging, as you are not the most flexible of doshas. Be patient with yourself, and it will come.

A NOTE ABOUT CORPSE POSE

Corpse Pose, or Savasana, is perhaps the most important pose for all three doshas. This pose incorporates the entire yoga routine deep into your bones, muscles, and tissues—as well as the mind. Don't skip it or skimp on the time. Give Savasana sufficient time at the end of your yoga practice. For Vata, 15 to 20 minutes is most beneficial. For Pitta, 10 to 15 minutes works well, and for Kapha, 5 to 10 minutes will do.

Pitta should avoid yoga at the hottest time of day, so schedule your classes accordingly. Pitta needs to let go of heat during their routine. Inversions create heat, especially in the head, so avoid those. Open chest poses and hip openers are great for Pitta. Try Camel Pose, Bow Pose, Bridge Pose, and Cobra Pose.

The breath should be steady and relaxed. You can even practice Cooling Breath (see page 117) to cool down between poses. Take your time in Corpse Pose. Cool down and relax for a good 10 to 15 minutes.

Kapha Yoga Guidelines

Oh, Kapha, how you love to do gentle, slow yoga, seated poses, forward bends, and twists. But resist the urge to slow down and luxuriate in your naturally well-lubricated body and get up and get moving! Warm up and limber your body before going into your routine. Stand tall and hold your poses for at least one minute. Get those arms over your head. Open your chest, bend backward, and feel the energy. If music helps you move faster, then by all means listen to it.

Breathe deeply during your routine, and don't be afraid if you get out of breath. Breathe rapidly (through your nose) and deeply at a steady rate. Move with more speed than Vata and Pitta between poses, but stay conscious and aware of your movements to avoid getting hurt. Create heat in your body, and even challenge yourself a bit.

Kapha does great practicing yoga during Kapha time of day, 6 a.m. to 10 a.m. This will help you begin your day with motivation and energy, and help keep you more energized and motivated throughout the day. Try cleansing and energizing Bellows Breath (see page 118), at the beginning or end of your routine, after Corpse Pose (page 104). Kapha benefits most from a shorter Corpse Pose, about 5 to 10 minutes.

YOGA POSES WITH DOSHIC MODIFICATIONS

Mountain Pose (Tadasana)

Once you have mastered this pose, so many other tasks in your life will feel less stressful. You can practice this while brushing your teeth, working at your job (if it requires standing on your feet), standing in line, washing dishes, and before meditation. When you are properly aligned, it should feel effortless, as if you can hold this pose forever without stress or strain. It will be as if a thread is attached to the crown of your head lifting you upward, increasing a sense of lightness and ease, and your feet will feel balanced and attached to the earth.

1. Stand with your feet together and parallel, arms loose by your sides, with palms facing forward, next to your thighs. Keep your gaze soft and forward. Your ears should be aligned over your shoulders. Allow your chest to open, and keep your shoulders back and down, with the shoulder blades gliding down your back, gently holding your spine, with a slight arch in your back. Your knees should be over your toes. Take special notice of your pelvis. It should be in a neutral position—not too far back or

too far forward. Move around a bit to find this point. Your neck should be long and natural.

2. Try to balance on all four corners of your feet: under the big toe, the pinky toe, the left side of your heel, and the right side of your heel. You can even lift your toes up to better feel this grounding, then slowly lower your toes. Close your eyes and feel your body sinking and grounding, and be still.

3. Open your eyes. On the inhale, ground the pose through your feet, calves, knees, and thighs. Feel the thighs pull toward one another as if you are holding a block between your upper thighs. Lengthen your tailbone downward. Feel your shoulders move down. Fill your rib cage with air and expand your torso.

4. On the exhale, extend from the sacrum through the spine and lengthen, feeling your torso contract. Feel the crown of your head open and connect to the universe. You can slightly tuck your chin on the exhale.

5. Keep your arms, hands, and fingers relaxed. Do the same with your face, neck, and throat.

6. Take at least 10 breaths, grounding and lengthening on the inhale, and contracting and realigning on the exhale.

DOSHA TIP: For Vata, focus on the inhale as a way to still the mind and ground the body. Breaths should be long and smooth. For Pitta, focus on finding quiet within, taking long breaths and feeling a mental and physical lift in the pose. Practice with eyes closed if you like. For Kapha, focus on lifting and expanding. Feel your muscles as you pay attention to each part of your body on the inhale and exhale. Breathing should be steady.

Down Dog (Adho Mukha Svanasana)

Do as the dogs do! Our three canine girls (one rescued from India) do their down dog poses every morning when they wake up—so should you. It's a great way to get blood moving to the head to create awareness, and to stretch and open the spine after a good night's sleep. Play with your dog pose, move around, bend your knees, and work your heels toward the floor. The first Down Dog of the day should be playful and flexible. Have fun with it. Down Dog can be looked at as a resting pose between more vigorous movements. For added strength and length, you can move easily between Plank and Down Dog. It's great for your core and can be a real workout in itself.

1. Begin the pose on all fours with your knees under your hips, spread hip-distance apart (which is usually closer than you think). Turn your toes under so the soles of your feet are facing out. Keep your arms straight, the insides of your elbows facing each other, your palms flat on the floor, and your fingers spread wide, with special attention to the middle finger knuckle, grounding you. Your hands should be shoulder-width apart or slightly closer. Your face should be facing toward the floor with your spine long and natural. Your knees are slightly behind the sit bones (the bones you sit on under the flesh of your buttocks) to facilitate lift.

2. To prepare your body, do a few Cat and Cow Poses (see page 97) a few times to loosen your spine.

3. On the inhale, with curled toes, push yourself up, lifting your knees off the floor, lifting from your hips, lengthening your torso, and straightening your arms. Straighten your legs and bring your heels toward the floor if possible (or just think about it!). Your knees can be slightly bent if that is more comfortable. Let your head hang and gaze toward your navel if that stretch feels good. If not, look back toward your feet. Soften your face.

4. On the exhale, lengthen and lift your hips, sinking deeper into the pose, and relax. Feel free to wiggle around and loosen up a bit, bending your knees and adjusting your arms. Find your center—especially on the first Dog of the day. On the inhale, feel your body getting longer and lighter. On the exhale, ground deeper.

5. Begin by holding the pose for 20 to 30 seconds. Work up to 60 seconds.

6. To come down, bend your knees on an exhale to the floor and sit back on your folded thighs, with the top of your toes against the floor. Sit on your heels. Alternatively, you can fold down into Child's Pose (see page 100).

DOSHA TIP: For Vata, move slowly between each round, breathe deeply, and extend your body through your arms and the feet, feeling your torso expand and extend. Hold for longer periods. For Pitta, feel the stretch in your torso and your arms and legs. Feel the cooling air filling your body by breathing through your nose. Hold the pose for shorter periods of time and rest in Child's Pose between repetitions. Kapha can do more repetitions at a faster pace and can hold the pose longer. Feel yourself lift, lengthen, and extend. Rest by sitting on your heels.

Tree Pose (Vrikasana)

Did you know that balance poses are just as good for your brain as they are for your body? The brain shifts from one area to another as you work in the balance pose, strengthening and creating new patterns and neural networks. Anytime you feel sluggish in your mind, do a Tree Pose or another balancing pose you like, and notice how it wakes you up.

1. Begin as you would in Mountain Pose (see page 94) and take a few deep grounding breaths. Looking straight ahead, on the inhale, slowly shift your weight to your right leg and feel the weight from your hip to the sole of your foot. On the exhale, lift your left leg and place your left foot firmly on the inside of the right thigh, below the knee or at the ankle—whichever is comfortable for you. You can even use your hand to help lift your foot and put it in place. Your pelvis should be neutral and your hips level with the ground. Your left leg is open and your knee is open to the side. I find it helpful to push my thigh into my foot for added balance.

2. If needed, stand next to a wall for balance. If you are not next to a wall, open your hands so your palms are facing forward. Slowly begin to raise your straight arms out to the side and then overhead. Turn your palms to face each other above your head. Breathe slowly and steadily, staring straight ahead. Your shoulders should be down and relaxed with your inner arms next to your ears.

3. On the inhale, feel the balance and adjust. On the exhale, lengthen your spine upward. Keeping your tailbone extended downward and your shoulders down, extending your fingers upward.

4. To come down, gracefully lower your arms and leg at the same time and place your foot lightly on the floor. Position yourself in Mountain Pose again, and then shift your weight to your left foot, and follow the same routine.

5. Hold each side for as long as comfortable.

DOSHA TIP: For Vata, take long, deep breaths, envision shooting roots deep into the ground through your feet, and be still with long, raised arms. For Pitta, feel light and cool in the pose, not rigid or straining. Be flexible. For Kapha, do several repetitions on either side. Feel your muscles moving up, and hold the balance. Ground with your feet, but reach up with your hands.

Cat Pose (Marjariasana) and Cow Pose (Bitilasana)

These two poses are performed together, so you may see this referred to simply as Cat-Cow Pose. Both work to stretch the lower spine and hips, and open the chest.

1. Come down to the floor on all fours with your palms flat on the ground, fingers spread, wrists lined up under your shoulders, and the insides of the elbows facing each other. Avoid hunching or shrugging your shoulders. The tops of your feet should be flat on the ground. Keep your knees hip-width apart. (Place a blanket or extra mat under your knees if this is uncomfortable.)

2. Take a few deep breaths and level out your back so your spine is straight from your tailbone to the crown of your head, with shoulders relaxed and down. Your spine and neck should be in alignment. Look about 12 inches in front of you on the ground.

3. On the exhale, arch your back so it becomes concave and your belly moves toward the floor. Keep your arms straight (Cow).

4. On the inhale, round and lift your shoulders, tuck in your pelvis, and push up through your back toward the ceiling (Cat).

5. Move back and forth between Cat and Cow, following your breath in and out, a few times.

DOSHA TIP: This asana is good for all doshas as described. The deep breaths with the movement can remove excess Vata. Pitta will love the muscular workout of the belly. When done a little faster, it's a great warm-up for Kapha.

CURIOUS CAT

For added flexibility, try the Curious Cat move: On all fours with your back straight and your chin slightly tucked, look over your left shoulder and move your left hip slightly to the side, parallel with the floor. Hold for two breaths. Then turn your head to the right side, move your right hip, and take two breaths. Repeat twice on each side. Feel your pelvis sway from side to side as you gaze toward the same side. Your shoulders will automatically shift to the opposite side from your gaze.

Twisted Chair Pose (Parivrtta Utkatasana)

This is perfect for planes, trains, automobiles, and anywhere you find yourself sitting for an extended period of time. Of course, adding twist poses to your routine is great for your core and organs. Twists can actually squeeze toxins out of the organs to start them on their way out of the body.

1. Using a chair without armrests, sit sideways with your side to the back of the chair, feet flat on the floor, and ankles as close together as possible. Your spine should be erect, but not rigid. Keep your shoulders down and relaxed, away from your ears. Your neck should be long, and your belly relaxed and soft. Keep your pelvis neutral, and notice that your weight is even on the sit bones (the bones you sit on under the flesh of your buttocks).

2. Take hold of the back of the chair with both hands and turn toward the right. Look over your right shoulder with a soft gaze. Inhale and exhale slowly. On the inhale, increase the twist. On the exhale, lengthen your spine, rotating even deeper if possible.

3. Repeat on the opposite side.

DOSHA TIP: All twists are good for all three doshas. Just remember not to push yourself beyond where your body wants to go. A good guideline is to not twist your neck and to align your gaze so that it is parallel with your belly button.

Legs-up-the-Wall Pose (Viparita Karani)

This is an absolute must for your routine, especially if you travel or stand on your feet all day. The first thing I do when I get to my accommodations after traveling is find a spot on the floor (or the bed) to do this pose. This relieves swelling and pressure in the feet, ankles, and calves, while the pooling of the blood in your belly eases the nervous system and allows you to relax.

1. Find a wall space where you can easily swing your legs up without any obstacles in the way.

2. Sit with your right hip, knee, and calf parallel to the wall. Scoot the side of your butt so that it is flat against the wall. Then swing your legs up and around until they are against the wall above you.

3. Adjust yourself so that you feel comfortable to relax in this position for 5 or 10 minutes. You can have a pillow or rolled-up towel handy to place under your head or neck.

4. You can keep your feet straight up, flexing and pointing the toes and turning your ankles in circles. You can also open your legs wide by allowing them to slide down the wall toward your sides. If you are able, you can bring the soles of your feet together and rest in this position with your legs on the wall.

5. To come down, bend your knees to your chest and roll over to your right side and push yourself up slowly, keeping your head and gaze down. Slowly lift your head as you become seated. Take a moment or two before standing.

Child's Pose (Balasana)

A resting pose between asanas, as well as a pose of deep healing and calming, Child's Pose will help you ground your practice whenever you decide to use it—beginning, middle, or end. Take your time here to feel your breath, still your mind, and integrate your practice into your mind and body.

1. Come down to your knees with the tops of your feet flat against the floor, your knees together or knees wider apart, whichever is more comfortable. If this is uncomfortable, place a rolled-up towel or blanket under your ankles or under your knees.

2. Stretch both arms up over your head, elongating your spine and falling forward to the ground with your arms outstretched in front of you with your upper arms next to your ears.

3. Place your forehead on the ground, and close your eyes. You can use a rolled-up towel or yoga block to place under your forehead if the stretch is too deep for you. Tuck your chin and rest. Bring your chest forward to rest on your thighs. Alternatively, you can place your arms along your sides, with your palms facing upward.

4. Notice your breath and on each exhale allow yourself to sink deeper into the pose. Count to 10, or come up when you feel ready, by lifting your torso slowly and keeping your gaze down. Come to a seated position on your feet.

Bridge Pose (Depada Pidam)

As with our Ayurvedic practice, opposite actions balance the dosha. Bridge Pose moves the hips up in a way that is opposite the normal motion, creating balance in the body. By lifting and stretching, the body can open up and heal, move better, and feel more at ease.

1. Lie on the floor with your knees bent and your feet moved back toward your buttocks, hip-width apart. Allow your big toes to turn to face each other slightly, and make sure to keep your knees over your feet.

2. Feel the back of your head against the floor. Your arms should be straight out by your sides with your palms facing down. You can turn to the right, lift up, and slightly tuck your left shoulder under your back and do the same on your left side. This will give you extra lift in your pose.

3. Keeping your lower back neutral (this is very important), ground your feet into the floor and allow your tailbone and hips to effortlessly lift up. Your shoulders will help create a foundation for the pose.

4. On an exhale, lift your spine and feel the arch come into your upper body. Your palms remain flat on the floor, your neck is relaxed, and your lower back is neutral.

5. Continue to breathe as you hold the lift for 30 to 40 seconds.

6. To come down, on an inhale, slowly and with control, lower your back, one vertebrae at a time. Your tailbone will be the last to come down. Take a breath or two, relax, and lift again, gradually increasing the hold time.

DOSHA TIP: As with any pose, it's important to know yourself and your limits. Pitta tends to push themselves through even though they may feel pain. Vata can be scattered and imprecise. Kapha may skimp and shy away from the harder poses. Bridge Pose is a great pose to explore these feelings. Kapha should lift higher and hold longer. Pitta can take their time to explore the pose, and find a place of ease and lift. Vata can practice this slowly, increasing strength in the limbs and finding support in the lower back.

Wide-Legged Forward Bend (Padottanasana)

Just watch any child on the playground and you will see them falling forward, laughing, and resting with ease, and then just as quickly popping up and running on to the next thing. We all come to this pose effortlessly as a child, and then we forget to do it, so we lose it. But you don't have to. Thinking like a child can help you move deeper into this pose and hold it longer for maximum benefit.

1. Stand straight with your legs spread out about 4 to 5 feet apart, parallel to each other.

To make this a regular Forward Fold, follow the same described for Wide-Legged Forward Bend, but keep your feet hip-width apart instead of the wide-legged stance.

2. On an exhale, bend forward, leading with your head and feeling the lift in your sit bones (the bones you sit on under the flesh of your buttocks). If you are able to, place your hands on the floor, or if not, place several yoga blocks in front of you and place your hands on the blocks.

3. If you can reach the floor, bend your elbows inside your knees and allow the crown of your head to make contact with the floor. You may need to adjust the width of your feet to get there. Don't strain. Listen to your body.

4. You can lift your head and look up, feeling the stretch in your spine and lower back, and then move the head back down.

5. To come up, place both hands on your waist or hips, keeping your head down. On an exhale, slowly raise up one vertebrae at a time, chin to chest, saving the head for last.

6. Establish your balance, then jump or walk your feet back together. You may want to arch your back in the opposite direction upon rising to equalize the pose. Just lift your arms up over your head and effortlessly bend back, arching the spine on an inhale, come up and bend forward, swinging the arms with you, on the exhale.

DOSHA TIP: This is an excellent pose for reducing Pitta in a gentle way, allowing it to flow out and cool off as the pose is held. Vata does well here to feel the stillness and foundation provided by the wide-legged stance. Kapha will benefit from establishing strong legs, an open chest, and lift of the tailbone and torso. Kapha can move in and out of the pose more quickly than the other doshas.

Sun Salutation

This pose is typically repeated 12 times—one round contains the left leg lunge and repeated on the right side with the right side lunge. The number 12 is the number of signs in the zodiac, so we perform one for each sign, facing east to salute the sun, the biggest star in the galaxy.

1. Face east toward the rising sun. Stand in Mountain Pose (see page 94) with your hands in a prayer position. Focus your attention on your breath, feeling your heartbeat. Bring all of your awareness to the center of your chest, to your heart chakra, and just take a few moments here.

2. Stand at the front of your yoga mat with your feet slightly less than hip-width apart and parallel. Plant your feet and feel your entire body fall into alignment. Allow your arms to be at your sides, palms turned forward, chin slightly tucked, and shoulders down. Gaze forward.

3. On an inhale, raise your arms in a circle above your head, flowing from your sides to above your head, and bring the palms together over the crown of your head. Keep your elbows straight and your arms behind your ears with a slight arch in your back. Look up.

4. On an exhale, fall forward, bringing your arms down to the floor into a forward bend. Bend your knees if you need to and use yoga blocks if your hands don't reach the floor. Let your head and neck hang down, creating a long spinal extension. From this pose, lift your head and look up, bringing your hands to your knees.

5. On an inhale, move your head and hands back down toward the floor (or yoga blocks for your hands if you can't reach the floor), and lengthen your torso.

6. Exhale and step your right foot back into a lunge. Make sure your bent left knee is not over your left foot. It should be aligned with the heel, perpendicular to the floor. Bring your left thigh parallel to the floor. On the inhale, lean back through your right heel to support the pose. Lengthen and arch the torso, and lean forward over the left thigh. Gaze in front of you and lift the arms over your head.

7. On the exhale, bring your arms down, place your palms on the mat, and step your left foot to the back, parallel to the right foot for Down Dog (see page 95). Spread your fingers on the mat and plant your feet firmly. You can bend your knees and lift your heels if you need to. Lift your belly high, arch your back, and send your hips and buttocks back. Look down.

8. Inhale and bring your torso forward until your shoulders are over your wrists in a plank. Your arms will be perpendicular to the floor. Try not to let your upper back collapse between your shoulder blades: Press your elbows inward, separating the shoulder blades. Look down at the floor. Then exhale as you bring first knees, then chest, then chin down to the floor in a wavelike motion.

9. On the inhale, push yourself up, making sure not to constrict your lower back. Push up so that your head and chest lift off the mat (this is called Cobra Pose). The elbows can remain bent and on the floor, or lifted slightly, close to the body. Only lift yourself as far as comfortable. Do not strain or crunch your lower back. Gaze forward.

10. Come back down to the floor, before pushing yourself up on the inhale into a Down Dog (see page 95), and step your right leg forward to a lunge, exhaling as you do so. You can keep hands down on the mat, or take a moment to

find your balance and lift your arms straight above your head. If your arms are lifted, bring them back down to the mat and bring your left leg forward and fold into a forward bend, with both hands on the floor or yoga block, and your head down.

11. On the inhale, rise up, swing your arms over your head and greet the sun with a smile on your face, gazing upward.

12. Bring your gaze and hands down to eye level. Press your palms into a prayer position over your heart. Take a deep breath. Find your Mountain Pose (page 94).

13. Repeat from step 2, lunging to opposite sides. Practice as many rounds as feels comfortable for you from 2 to 12 rounds. Kapha, do one more. Pitta, do one less. Vata, stay where you feel comfortable.

DOSHA TIP: Kapha can add a little speed to the routine, maybe hopping or jumping to switch feet in the lunges. Vata can perform the movements more slowly, concentrating on an easy flow and proper alignment. Ground your hips toward the mat on the lunges for a more stable posture. Pitta, while you have the urge to power through, try to feel each stretch in your arms, legs, and spine. Make sure to breathe with each pose, slow down, and feel the whole body workout.

Corpse Pose (Savasana)

Simply put, this is your most important pose. Pitta usually wants to skip out before it happens, Kapha falls asleep, and Vata finds themselves cold. But with the proper preparation, you will find that this pose will help you integrate your entire practice deep, deep down into the seven layers of tissues: plasma, blood, muscle, fat, bone, nervous system, and reproductive tissue. If you skip it, you are truly missing out on a full yoga asana practice. If you are doing this on your own, rather than in a class being led by an instructor, set a gentle timer to bring you out of the pose. This way, all you need to do is focus on relaxation.

1. Lie on the floor on your back with your legs stretched out long, legs slightly apart. Allow your feet to fall naturally to the sides.

2. Relax your shoulders away from your ears and feel your arms get heavy as they sink into the floor, palms facing up.

3. Allow the back of your neck to lengthen, and relax your face and jaw. Feel the back of your head sink into the floor.

4. Let your belly soften. Feel your lower back and pelvis release and remain neutral.

5. Do a body scan, beginning with your toes and then moving to the soles of your feet, your ankles, and so on. Moving up, as you focus on each body part, take a deep breath, and on the exhale, release any stress or tension in that area. Allow yourself to feel the sense of relaxation and letting go.

6. Feel your entire body melt into the floor. And just relax.

7. When you are ready to come out of the pose, begin by taking several deep breaths through your nose, expanding your belly on the inhale, and feeling your belly button fall back toward your spine on the exhale. Begin to wiggle your fingers and toes. Feel free to bend your knees. When you feel ready, roll over to your left side and use your hands and arms to push up, allowing your head to rise up last, into a seated position.

DOSHA TIP: Vata can get set up with a blanket, an eye covering, and perhaps a folded or rolled-up blanket to support the neck, feet, and knees. Pitta does well with an eye covering to help slow down, go within, and be still. Feel free to use blankets as supports as needed. Kapha does best lying directly on the floor or mat without props or support, but do use them if needed.

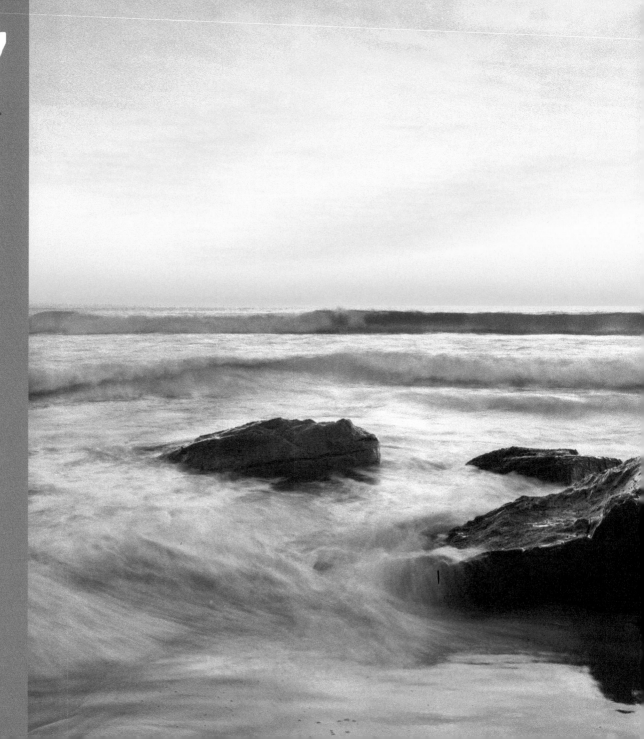

CHAPTER 7

Spiritual Rituals
and Practices

The words *spirituality* and *religion* are often placed in the same sentence, but it doesn't have to work that way. You can have a deep spiritual side and not be religious at all. Or you can be religiously observant but not feel especially spiritual. And you can certainly be both. It's a personal matter, but a spiritual practice can connect you to your inner self and others, if you choose.

For the most part, we live in a Vata society. What this means is that we are constantly bombarded by distractions—smartphone alerts, televisions and computer screens, noise from the radio, magazines, billboards, navigation systems, and so on. Once, at an Ayurvedic conference when I was feeling particularly "zen," I floated onto an elevator only to be confronted by a screen blaring news at me that I didn't want to know as I descended ten floors. This isn't an anomaly. It's hard to find moments of quiet and stillness in our daily life. So we have to create them, find time for them, be imaginative, and be insistent on taking a break from the daily grind. Learning to be playful, kicking off your shoes, and staring off into space is a great way to begin.

In Ayurveda, there are many rituals that can help us feel a purpose and a deeper connection to the path. You can do all or none—it's up to you. In this chapter, you will find a few ways we connect ourselves on a deeper spiritual level to this ancient practice.

COOKING WITH MINDFULNESS

When preparing and cooking food, try to be fully present and engage all your senses. When you are fully present, the sounds, smells, and sight of the food you are preparing will offer clues about when to add the next ingredient, when to take the food off the heat, and how to combine it with other foods. As you cook with mindfulness, you will soon begin to cook by feel rather than by following a recipe. The food will "speak" to you, and your senses will let you know what is needed. And in this way, your food will nourish all of your senses.

When I learned Ayurvedic cooking with Amadea Morningstar, she taught us to chant while preparing food, to infuse the meal with deep healing wisdom and ourselves with feelings of well-being. Physically connecting to the preparation of your food begins the digestive process, and you will be able to more fully assimilate the meal when you begin to eat. The digestive "fires" are stoked just by cooking the meal and observing the alchemy taking place.

Tips for Cooking with Mindfulness

- As you cook, chant, *"om tare tuttare ture mama ayur jnana punye pustim kuru svaha,"* which is a chant to the Buddhist Goddess of Compassion, White Tara. The chant is a means to liberation from disease, fear, and disturbing thoughts, creating a path for health and well-being.

- Dress in all white, if you'd like, to formalize your practice and honor the importance of the cooking. The color white represents purity.

- Remove all the distractions from your kitchen. Turn off the television and radio, put your smartphone on silent, and wait on the wine. You must pay attention when cooking to really connect to the food and the process of cooking.

- Invite friends over to cook. Instead of idle chitchat in the kitchen, join together for a round of chanting to connect you all to the food and align your beings before you eat together.

- Consider using utensils and pots and pans for the season (silver for summer, brass or copper for winter). Silver is "cooling"; brass and copper are "heating."

MANTRA CHANTING

Chanting mantras can have a soothing effect on your mind and body, and there are even studies being done now to show how certain sounds and syllables, when chanted, can create physical changes to promote well-being and elevate moods.

Mantra literally means "mind tool" or "vehicle for focus and concentration." Don't confuse a mantra with an affirmation: affirmations are used to set an intention, while a mantra is used for focus and concentration. The meaning of the mantra you chant isn't necessary to know; rather, it is the vibrational essence of the sounds that align you with your practice. The following are a few guidelines for each dosha:

Vata—warm, soothing, soft, and calming sounds. Mantras should be chanted silently, as chanting out loud can increase Vata energy and may be depleting. Try just a minute or two out loud and then switch to silently repeating the mantra in your head. Best choices are *Ram*, *Hoom*.

Pitta—cooling, calming, soothing, sweet sounds. Mantras can be sung out loud or mentally. If out loud, keep your voice calm, cool, and steady. Best choices are *Aum*, *Aim*, *Shrim*, *Sham*.

Kapha—stimulating, warming, and active sounds. Sing out loud in a robust, cheerful manner. Best choices are *Hoom*, *Aum*, *Aym*.

You can chant these sounds to set the stage for meditation practice, when you are feeling anxious or nervous, during everyday activities, or virtually anytime, really. They help the mind relax and detoxify the same way meditation does. Mantras keep you in the moment, which is the most relaxing place to be.

CHAKRA CHANTING

The *chakras* (pronounced with a hard *ch* like in the word *change*) are said to be seven spinning wheels of energy that move along our spine from our root chakra at the base of the spine, to the crown chakra at the center of the top of the head. These wheels relate to different emotional and physical centers of our body, and have vibrant colors, harmonious sounds, and deep connections to the soul.

Chanting the sounds of the chakras, called toning, while visualizing their places and colors can have a powerful healing effect. You may notice that you have an area of the body where you repeatedly have issues—like headaches, an achy lower back, menstrual cramps, or hoarseness of your throat. We would say that area is calling for your attention, and chakra chanting might be the healing you need. However, you should do the chanting for each chakra to promote balance in them all.

Root Chakra (Muladhara)

The root chakra grounds us. It is our home base, our survival instincts, and a place of safety and security. A tree, in order to grow and expand toward the universe, must have a healthy, sturdy root system. So must we. When the root chakra is balanced, we feel safe and sound, self-assured, steady, and strong. When out of balance, we can feel unstable, groundless, foundationless, nervous, fearful, and scared as if we don't have ground to stand on, as if our basic needs are not being met.

Physically, the root chakra covers the area from the lowest point of your groin (the perineum) down through the hips, thighs, and legs to the soles of your feet.

To balance this chakra, visualize a swirling ball of red at the base of your spine in both the front and back body. See the ball swirling clockwise along the root to cleanse, hold strong, and offer safety and security. As you do this, chant the sound of the root chakra: *Lam. Lam. Lam.*

Sacral Chakra (Svadhisthana)

As we move up the body, we come to the second chakra, the area from your genitals to just below your navel. This is an area of passion, sexuality, emotions, and creativity. Through this chakra, we experience the sensuality of the world. When balanced, we feel connected to others on many levels, we are able to give and receive (pleasure and emotions), we are expressive and fluid, and we are secure in our sexuality, sensuality, creativity, and movement.

Imbalance in the sacral chakra can inhibit us, cause fear of commitment and expression of our needs, create insecurity and lack of libido, and cause us to feel stuck and/or unsure.

To balance this chakra, visualize a swirling ball of orange below your belly button, bright and vibrant and self-assuring. As you do this, chant the sound of the sacral chakra: *Vam. Vam. Vam.*

Solar Plexus Chakra (Manipura)

Just above the belly button, the solar plexus chakra rules the center of your torso, your belly. This is your ego, your identity, your center of people, power, and possessions—your personality. This is your expression of self, will, desires, and intellect. When balanced, this chakra regulates our feelings of power and expression. We feel confident, open, and easy-going with our thoughts, plans, and outlook on life. We move forward easily, and often people will follow our bright light.

When out of balance, the ego can spiral out of control. Blame abounds. Suspicion of motivations can lead to wrecked relationships. There is a feeling of loss, obsession, and manipulation.

To balance this chakra, visualize a swirling ball of blazing yellow like the sun shining in your belly—a light for all to see. As you do this, chant the sound of the solar plexus chakra: *Ram. Ram. Ram.*

Heart Chakra (Anahata)

Located in the center of your chest is your center of compassion, forgiveness, unconditional love, and awareness. One of the most important aspects of the heart chakra is love of self, forgiveness of self, acceptance of self, and compassion for self. Once you have truly mastered these, your heart chakra has the infinite capability of offering all these blessings to others. The well never runs dry. The more self-acceptance you have, the more you can offer that to others. This offers a deep sense of connection, unity, peace, and love.

When out of balance, the heart chakra feels closed to giving and receiving. Old wounds fester and the heart aches; we cannot forgive and forget. We feel jealousy instead of joy, pain instead of pleasure.

To balance the heart chakra, visualize a swirling ball of emerald green around your heart. Imagine your chest filling up with this green ocean of love and forgiveness, gently swirling, building energy, and moving out into the world. As you do this, chant the sound of the heart chakra: *Yam. Yam. Yam.*

Throat Chakra (Vishuddha)

Found at the base of the throat, the thyroid gland, and up and around the ears to the back of the head, this chakra is not only about true self-expression—speaking your truth—but also about listening and discernment. Listening is often more important than speaking. Those with a balanced throat chakra know when to be quiet and when to speak up. When balanced, the voice may be melodious, fluid, and mellifluous. We know how to hear what is being said and decide for ourselves what the truth is, and we know what best serves us and will not be persuaded otherwise by excessive talk from others.

When out of balance, we may be shy, timid, and have trouble speaking up for ourselves. We believe everything we hear with no sense of discernment. Or we may talk incessantly without noticing that no one is listening.

To balance the throat chakra, visualize a swirling ball of turquoise blue in the area of the throat, ears, and the back of the head. As you do this, chant the sound of the throat chakra: *Hum. Hum. Hum.*

Third Eye Chakra (Ajna)

Located on the forehead between the eyebrows, the third eye chakra is also often called the brow chakra. It is the center of intuition, connection to self, psychic abilities, vision, and perception. When balanced, this chakra leads us not only to inner realms, but also to the outer realms of the universe, where we feel a sense of connection to all of creation: a knowingness that is hard to describe, but nevertheless moves us into a place of subtle energy where everything is possible. Meditation while visualizing this area can lead you to a state of pure bliss, light, and unlimited potentialities.

When out of balance, we find it difficult to get a clear vision of ourself and our place in the world; we experience a dullness in perception or feel out of touch with reality. We have difficulty making decisions. We feel stuck with the way things are and have no sense of the way things could be.

To balance the third eye chakra, visualize a swirling ball of indigo arising behind your third eye—your forehead between your eyebrows. As you do this, chant the sound of the third eye chakra: *Sham. Sham. Sham.*

Crown Chakra (Sahasrara)

Known as the thousand-petal lotus, the crown chakra, at the center of your head or just above, connects you to the universe and infinite possibilities for your being. When we are connected to this chakra, we notice an increased sense of awareness, a connection to all beings—sentient and nonsentient. We have a deep sense of the limitlessness of the universe. We are unbounded awareness itself—blissful. We have the knowledge that there is no separation between ourselves and everything else in the universe. We are infinite, boundless, pure awareness, connected to all.

When out of balance, our blissful sense of connection is lost. We feel adrift, unsure, and untethered. Our minds are closed to the infinite possibilities around us. We may become disconnected, withdrawn, and isolated.

To balance the crown chakra, visualize a crown of pure white or violet light around your head and feel it pour down your body and surround you. As you do this, chant the sound of the crown chakra (called the *Bijah*, or seed), the sound of the universe, the first sound ever made: *Om. Om. Om.*

BREATH WORK (PRANAYAMA)

While you may hear pranayama referred to simply as "breathing exercises," the formal definition of this Sanskrit term is the conscious control of the breath through specific techniques and exercises, or breath work. Prana is the life force that flows through all sentient beings, and the great Hindu sages of Ayurveda discovered that many different types of breath retention and flow could change our physiology as well as help balance the doshas. They also believed that the regulation of the breath can decrease illness and increase one's life span.

You may notice when you begin doing breath work that one or the other nostril is clogged. This is nothing to be concerned about. The sinuses are made of tissue that is erectile, meaning that it fills with blood and then drains over time. This usually happens about every 90 minutes—you will notice that at any one time either the left or right side is more open, depending on blood flow.

There are no tools or equipment or fancy clothes or shoes needed to practice pranayama. All you need is a comfortable place to sit and a little bit of time. You might want to have a box of tissues handy in case you need to blow your nose. It's best to practice pranayama on an empty stomach if possible.

For all breath work, make sure you are seated in a comfortable position—on the floor, in a chair, or on a bed. Sit in a fashion (such a cross-legged) so that your chest is open and that you have room to move your arms. Your spine should be erect but not rigid. For some of the breath work, you can place your tongue at the "fire point"—the ridge behind your front teeth—when you begin your practice. Just allow your tongue to float up and rest in this position. It will take stress off your jaw, prevent you from clenching your teeth, and also create balance, which is an added benefit.

At the end of all breath work, take a few minutes to let your breathing return to normal before moving on to another activity. Notice how your mind and body feel. Do you feel grounded? Cooler? Hotter? Be aware, and take note. Making pranayama part of your daily routine takes just a few minutes a day, but has enormous benefits.

Alternate Nostril Breathing (Nadi Shodhana)

Healing for all doshas, particularly Vata

Pranayama for grounding, relief from anxiety and worry

One of my teachers calls this type of breath work the king of all pranayama, and I can understand why. It both calms the mind and invigorates the body by creating an open state of conscious awareness. By breathing air into one nostril and out the other, you are creating an endless loop around the line of the chakras called the *sushumna*, thereby balancing your masculine and feminine sides. With each deep

inhale, you oxygenate your blood, and with each exhale, you relax deeper, while ridding the body of stress and anxiety. Among all its healing benefits, it may help relieve a headache, and it is believed by some to lessen hot flashes in menopausal women when practiced at least 15 minutes a day.

Take it slow and feel the qualities of the breath on each inhale and exhale.

1. Prepare by touching the index finger and the middle finger of your right hand to your palm, keep your thumb up and your ring finger and pinky open (they don't have to be uncomfortably extended). This hand position is called the *vishnu mudra*. You will begin by using the thumb of your right hand to gently close off your right nostril. Your ring finger will also come into play in step 3 when it is time to close off the left nostril. (An alternate hand position is to place your index and middle finger between your eyebrows so that you can use your thumb and ring finger to close off your nostrils as described in the following steps.)

2. Close off your right nostril with your thumb. Inhale through your left nostril deeply all the way down to your pelvic floor. Exhale up through your torso to your throat and let the breath out through your left nostril, keeping your thumb in place.

3. Inhale deeply again and, at the end, or top, of the inhale, close your left nostril with your

> During alternate nostril breathing, you may experience a cessation of thought, stillness of body, and deep relaxation of the nervous system. When your body is in this state, it can naturally begin the healing process. It is only when relaxed that the body can perform the functions of cleansing, repair, and rejuvenation. Doing this breath work can help you reach that state on a regular basis.

right ring finger. Open your thumb on the right nostril and exhale. At the bottom of the exhale, pause for a moment, and then inhale deeply again through the right nostril.

4. Close your right nostril again with your thumb, and exhale left. Now inhale left, close, and exhale right.

5. Continue breathing this way—right and left—for 20 breaths. Each inhale and exhale is one breath. You can use your left hand to count the breaths. When you have gone through your fingers two times, you have completed your session. Build up the number of breaths you do in a session slowly. (Very advanced practitioners may do as many as 108 breaths!)

ADVANCED TIP: Another way to practice to increase stillness in the mind and body during alternate nostril breathing is to hold your breath between the inhale and exhale. This pause is called *kumbhaka*. When you feel the urge to swallow or you reach a count of 16 seconds, release the hold. Avoid this pause if you have high blood pressure, pulmonary problems, or a migraine.

MANTRA TIP: You can silently practice the mantra *So Hum* during alternate nostril breathing. On the in breath, silently say "So" to yourself. If you pause as described in the earlier tip, say, "O." On the out breath say, "Hum."

Cooling Breath (Sheetali)

Pitta reducing

Pranayama for cooling and calming the mind and body; reduces blood pressure

While this is great breath work for Pitta, it's good anytime you feel overheated, mentally or physically. It's also great for women who are experiencing hot flashes. This one even works well while driving in your car where overheating emotionally can happen! If you are doing it in your car, though, keep your eyes on the road and your hands on the wheel.

1. Sit comfortably, keeping your spine erect but not rigid. Place your hands comfortably on your lap with the palms facing up. Take one or two deep breaths in and out through your nose.

2. If you are able, roll your tongue and stick it out of your mouth just a bit. (If you can't roll your tongue, see the tip accompanying this exercise.) Now inhale through your mouth, pulling the air in through the loop in your tongue, filling your chest and belly. This should feel cool and calming, and will fill your torso with air.

3. Withdraw your tongue back into your mouth, and place the tip of your tongue at the "fire point"—the ridge behind your front

teeth. Exhale fully through your nose. As you exhale, feel stress, frustration, and heat leaving the body.

4. Stick your tongue out again and repeat this process 10 times.

TIP: If you can't roll your tongue, either purse your lips and suck the air in that way, or widen your lips like an exaggerated smile and pull air in through the sides of the mouth through the cheeks (this is called *sheetkari*, or hissing breath). Exhale as described in the exercise.

Bellows Breath (Bhastrika)

Kapha reducing

Pranayama for firing up metabolism and waking up the body

Bellows Breath is a heating breath that opens the lungs, promotes digestion, eliminates toxins, increases oxygen intake, boosts the metabolism, and creates a sense of feeling "fired up." Begin slowly. Make sure you are capable of full belly breathing before trying this practice. If in doubt, leave it out.

This is a very active pranayama designed to get the blood flowing and mind working. The Bellows Breath requires force exerted from your diaphragm to exhale—pushing the air up and out—and a quick passive inhale. Some people even break a sweat doing this heating breath.

Do not practice Bellows Breath if you are pregnant or menstruating, or if you have heart problems or respiratory ailments. Also, avoid this breath if you have high blood pressure, ulcers, severe gastrointestinal problems, or a hernia.

1. If you are sitting on a chair, scoot forward until you are seated on the edge, keeping your spine erect but not rigid as for all pranayama. Place your hands on your belly or on your thighs.

2. Take two or three deep belly breaths to begin, expanding your belly on the inhale like a balloon and pulling your belly button back toward your spine on the exhale.

3. Take another breath and exhale by forcing out the air on your exhale, using your diaphragm. Your in breaths will be passive, and will happen naturally as your body takes the air back in.

4. Do 10 breaths in this fashion, beginning slowly, and, as you get acclimated to it, pick up speed. At the tenth breath on the inhalation, hold your breath before expelling it slowly and resting.

TIP: During this breath work, you might feel that your abdomen and chest move in an exaggerated fashion. This is normal.

MEDITATION

There are many different types of meditation, but you don't need to go searching just yet. In this section, you'll find instructions for how to meditate. Stick with this process for your 21-day plan before trying a practice you think will be better for you. We have a tendency to look here and there, constantly searching for something better, or doubting our choices. If, after 21 days, you'd like to find a teacher, an app, or a group that teaches something different, that's fine. But do stick with it. You will find wisdom not only there—but within.

Some of the biggest misconceptions about meditation are that it's really hard, it's too difficult to sit still, and it's necessary to completely clear your mind of thoughts. Here's the thing: It's not too hard when you use a good method and receive instruction. When you know how to sit properly with support, you should be able to maintain that posture for 5 to 20 minutes at least. And you will never clear your mind of thoughts. So there you go! But you will find that the thoughts quiet down, take a back seat, and slowly begin to fade away.

Three main things happen when we meditate: (1) we have thoughts, (2) we get sleepy, and (3) we feel still and quiet. We find ourselves in that place of stillness for a moment, and then we have a thought. So we start again—again and again.

Meditation is about learning to work with your thoughts. I tell my meditation students that the second you notice you are thinking, you are meditating! For a change, you are in control of your mind, rather than your mind being in control of you. We watch our thoughts arise, and we choose to let them go. Like clouds in the sky, we cannot grasp them, cling to them, pull them down, and examine them. We simply watch them go by—peacefully, calmly, letting go over and over again.

If you find yourself getting sleepy during meditation, it is usually an indication that you are not getting enough sleep—it's that simple. So get a better night's rest so that you can

> One of my meditation teachers, Davidji, taught us to use the acronym *RPM* to remember some very sound advice: Rise. Pee. Meditate. This truly is great advice! Before you become distracted by the upcoming day, get up, take care of your body's needs, and then find a comfortable seat and start your meditation practice.

meditate well. If you do get sleepy while meditating, just open your eyes, and take a deep breath. Remind yourself that you are meditating and gently close your eyes again.

It can be useful to work with a mantra to help you focus. I use the mantra *So Hum* with my students. This can be translated as "I Am" in Sanskrit, but it is truly the vibrational quality of the sound of *So Hum* that can lull your brain into that peaceful place of unconditional love, acceptance, and forgiveness.

To practice meditation:

1. Set a timer for your desired length of meditation to avoid being distracted by checking the clock during your practice. Allow a few extra minutes for steps two through five, as you prepare yourself to meditate.

2. Find a comfortable position so that you won't be distracted by your body. You may be most comfortable propped up in bed with a bunch of pillows behind your back, on the floor on a meditation cushion, or on your favorite chair. Take some time figuring out what works best for you. Lying down is not advised, especially for beginners, because it is too close to the position we get in to go to sleep.

3. Your spine should be erect but not rigid. Relax your shoulders and arms. Place your palms up or down on your lap or thighs. Your pelvis should be in a neutral position—not too far back or too far forward. Keep your neck straight with your chin slightly tucked. Relax your face and jaw. Placing your tongue at the "fire point," the ridge behind your front teeth, will help relax your jaw.

4. Once you are in this position, notice if you are holding tension in any area of your body. If so, gently flex that area, and then relax. You can also breathe into that area by focusing on it as you inhale, and then relaxing it as you exhale.

5. Practice five rounds of Alternate Nostril Breathing (see page 116) or take a few deep belly breaths. Allow your belly to soften and expand on the inhale, and on the exhale, contract the belly button to bring it back toward your spine. Settle into your body.

6. Notice any sounds or smells. Also notice the temperature. Acclimate yourself to your surroundings. Incorporate them into your meditation so that you will not be distracted by them. Simply notice and let go.

7. Silently begin to repeat the mantra *So Hum*: "So" on the in breath and "Hum" on the out breath. If you get mixed up, that's okay; it is the intention that matters.

8. If your mind begins to wander, notice that you are thinking, and then gently and kindly nudge yourself back to your mantra. *So Hum.*

9. Continue this way for 5 to 20 minutes, or longer if possible.

My Meditation Journey

I have had extraordinary opportunities in my life to meditate with some of the greatest living teachers. I began a meditation practice when I was 28 years old and living in Israel. I sat in the living room of an Israeli couple who had just returned from India. Our small group did yoga asanas, and then we sat in meditation. The instruction was in Hebrew, but the meditation was Hindu. I found I was a natural at sitting still for long periods of time. It must have been all the Kapha in me! As I continued practicing, I grew excited by the benefits I was experiencing.

Later, in the United States, I continued my practice, sitting with a Jewish meditation group, Shambhala Meditation, and eventually I began Buddhist meditation. For many years, I attended silent meditation retreats at the Gaia House in England, the Insight Meditation Society, and the Barre Center for Buddhist Studies in Barre, Massachusetts. I sat in retreats with Christopher Titmuss, Charles Genoud, Gregory Kramer, Lama Surya Das, Sharon Salzberg, Joseph Goldstein, Jack Kornfield, Christina Feldman, Deepak Chopra, David Simon, and many more amazing teachers.

When I began my Ayurvedic studies, I learned about Vedic Meditation, Transcendental Meditation (TM), and other Hindu practices. I have taken all these practices and all the mantras I received and put them together in my own unique expression of meditation.

As with yoga, I find that the longer you practice, the more you are able to trust your own mind and discover for yourself what best serves you. I encourage you to dig deep into your practice, find a teacher, go on retreats, and turn your meditation into your own—but practice, practice, practice. The result? Pure happiness.

10. When the timer rings, release your mantra (i.e., stop repeating it), but keep your eyes closed for a few minutes.

11. Take a deep breath in through your nose, down into your belly, and then slowly let it go. Notice the changes in your body and mind as you shift from a meditative state of consciousness to a more waking state of consciousness.

12. When you are ready, slowly open your eyes. Take your time shifting into your day. Try not to race off to the next task. Keep the treasures of your meditation practice with you as you go about your daily activities. You can always return to that stillness and silence just by being still, breathing, and repeating the mantra.

TIP: During meditation, it's possible you may experience complex emotions, disturbing thoughts, unsettling memories, body aches and pains, and more. If this happens, try to let go of each occurrence as it arises, just as you would with wandering thoughts. As you become more skilled, which will take time, or begin working with a teacher, you can learn how to work with those feelings, thoughts, and emotions in a way that will enrich your well-being and help you become happier and more peaceful. If something disturbing comes up during meditation and nags at you later, feel free to reach out to a friend or teacher.

EARTHING

As a child, I couldn't wait to take off my shoes and run around on the grass after school. Those were the days before everyone was required to pick up their dogs' poop—so it was a precarious romp at times, but it was well worth it. Today, being barefoot on the earth actually has a name: earthing. People are finding that earthing offers many benefits, such as improved sleep, greater concentration and focus, and feelings of happiness. There are even earthing products you can buy, like a grass mat for under your desk. Nevertheless, I think you can get the most benefit by taking a break and walking outside as often as possible. Hopefully you have a park nearby or a backyard to wander around in barefoot. If not, take a drive and find a good spot.

In Ayurveda, balancing ourselves with the elements is one of the keys to good health. In fact, Ayurveda has a long history of connecting with the earth elements. The feel of the earth on the soles of your feet is rejuvenating, calming, and enlivening. Just thinking about it makes my toes wiggle with delight! If you remember being a child playing outside in warm weather, you probably don't need much instruction here, but here are a few anyway with your dosha in mind.

To practice earthing:

1. Find a spot of grass, beach, or dirt path and remove your shoes.

2. Take a deep breath and ground yourself by feeling the earth under the soles of your feet, and under each toe.

3. Notice how it feels to shift your balance from one part of your foot to another.

4. Stand still for a few breaths, using all of your senses to notice how you feel.

5. Now take a walk. For Vata and Pitta, walk slowly and meditatively (i.e., allowing thoughts to come and go without trying to grasp on to them). For Kapha, walk with more purpose and a faster gait.

6. It's important to just notice how you feel. Empty your head and be present with the earth beneath your feet and the sky above your head.

Some people in India have made certain trees part of their daily rituals by walking around them in the morning, barefoot, of course. These trees, it turns out, give off healing chemicals that the people pick up as they walk around them. You might have a magic tree in your own backyard. For example, the bamboo palm, an air purifier, removes poisonous chemicals from the atmosphere, including benzene and formaldehyde. Other plants detox the air, too. Some of these include the peace lily, chrysanthemum, and aloe vera. So in addition to earthing, you can bring plants and trees into and around your home for their elemental benefits as well as their beauty.

SUN GAZING

Sun gazing is pretty much what it sounds like—gazing at the sun. However, there are some precautions to take: Don't stare at the sun for more than 10 seconds at a time, do so with an unfocused gaze (a soft, not intense, focus), and practice at sunrise and sunset, not when the sun is at its brightest.

The ancient rishis discovered that staring at the sun at sunrise and sunset infuses the body with unbounded energy and feelings of contentment and happiness. Perhaps it is because sunlight activates the pineal gland, sometimes referred to as the "God gland," triggering the release of two important hormones, serotonin and melatonin, among others. The sunlight also helps our bodies produce vitamin D, which is necessary for healthy skin and bones. Perhaps it's also the quality of earthing (see page 122) while sun gazing, which when combined with the practice can increase awareness and focus.

To practice sun gazing:

1. Check the time for sunrise or sunset in your area that day.

2. Go to a place outdoors just as the sun is rising or setting. It is okay if you cannot see the horizon. Simply facing east (at dawn) or west (at sunset) will still imbue you with the sun's energy.

3. Take off your shoes and ground your feet into the earth. Then sit or remain standing.

4. With an unfocused gaze, look toward the sun for no more than 10 seconds. Look away, and then repeat two or three times.

5. If you'd like to incorporate a mantra, try *om namah shivaya*, which I like for this practice. Silently repeat the mantra to yourself while gazing.

6. Take a moment to notice how you are feeling.

7. Give thanks to the sun for its presence.

FOOT WASHING AND OIL MASSAGE (KANSA VATKI)

After all that earthing (see page 122), it's a good idea to wash your feet before going to bed, if you don't have time for a shower or bath. Regardless, it is a lovely practice to rinse off the feet after a long day—it's refreshing, cooling, and healing, as many impurities can enter the body through the soles of the feet.

For this daily practice, I use warm water, a washcloth, and a soap with pumice in it. I personally use pumice soap from India called Gandhaali's Foot Scrub Soap, but any natural pumice soap will do. Alternatively, you can grind ¼ cup of adzuki beans in your spice grinder for a good pumice substitute; just add some water and 2 to 3 drops of tea tree oil to make a paste.

The traditional ritual of *kansa vatki* can actually take more than an hour, and involves a bowl made of copper, tin, and silver, and a kansa wand (a dome-shaped tool made from special metal) for deep massage of the Ayurvedic acupressure points (marma points). It's a lovely practice if you can set aside time for it, but for most of us, a simple foot oiling before bed, as described here, will have great benefits as well.

I usually oil my feet when I get into bed, but you might like to do it right after washing. The best oil to use is called bhringaraj oil. The herb bhringaraj is usually mixed in sesame seed oil, and is known for its calming and cooling actions. It's also a great herb for the scalp and hair; it is said to prevent premature graying as well as stimulate hair growth. (See the resources on page 161.)

Instructions for foot washing:

1. With a pair of socks nearby, sit on the side of the bathtub or fill a bowl with warm water.

2. Wash one foot at a time—between the toes, the soles of the foot, the ankle, and the top of the foot. Dry your feet thoroughly before going on to the next step.

3. Pour a small amount of oil (about the size of a dime) into the palm of your hand. Rub your hands together to warm up the oil.

4. Massage one foot at a time. Cover your foot with oil—from the toes and sole, to the top of the foot and the ankle. Like I do, you can take this opportunity to work on your "yoga toes"

by inserting four fingers through the spaces between your toes. Spread your fingers between your toes for a few moments.

5. Massage each toe from base to tip, and give each toe a little twist when you get to the top of the toe. Run your fingers firmly down the top of your foot, in the space between each toe, from the base of the toe all the way along the top of the foot.

6. Massage around the ankle, and using your palm, rapidly stroke the sole of foot several times, creating heat. Then using both palms, massage the sides of the foot the same way.

7. Using your thumbs, give yourself a pressure-point massage along the sole of the foot.

8. Put on your sock and repeat with the other foot. Then move on to head oiling (see below) to complete this evening routine.

HEAD OILING

Head oiling is an incredible technique that calms your mind, cools your body, and creates a deep sense of well-being. In combination with a foot massage, your nervous system relaxes deeply, allowing for a good night's sleep. Use the same oil as in the foot massage, bhringaraj oil (see the resources on page 161). Your hair should be dry when you perform head oiling.

Instructions for head oiling:

1. Pour a small amount of the oil (about the size of a quarter) into the palm of your hand, and then rub it onto the crown of your head and massage your scalp using the pads of your fingers for 2 to 3 minutes.

2. Massage the oil around your ears and the base of your neck. Dab your pinky in the oil and massage it into the inside of your ear as well.

3. Go to bed as usual; there should be no need for a towel since just a small amount of oil was used.

FOR A DEEPER EXPERIENCE:

1. Warm the oil by running the tightly capped bottle under hot water.

2. Pour about a tablespoon of the warm oil onto the crown of your head and massage your scalp using the pads of your fingers.

3. Work the oil through your hair.

4. Massage the oil around your ears and the base of your neck. Dab your pinky in the oil and massage it into the inside of your ear as well.

5. Cover your head with a towel for about 30 minutes or overnight. Sleep with a towel on your head or on your pillow.

TIP: For the first routine, use just enough oil to penetrate the scalp and send the amazing herb into the tissues of your scalp. The head massage itself is relaxing and should help you fall—and stay—asleep.

SEX

Sex is sacred. There is no doubt that intimate relationships are an important part of life and can be expressed in several ways, sex among them. Each dosha responds differently to sex, so it's important to know this and to know your partner's dosha to have the best sex life possible. The Ayurvedic text, *Ashtanga Hridayam*, offers details for sexual relations. While this text was based on the seasons and the food in India, we can use lessons from it today.

Ayurvedic texts state that sex depletes ojas, our life essence that feeds our vital energy, strength, and overall health. We want to make sure that we are healthy mentally and physically so that we have some ojas to expend. Before deciding to have sex, pay attention to your own levels of ojas. Notice if you feel weak, low energy, or depleted. If so, it may not be good for you to expend your energy on sex.

According to Ayurvedic texts, frequency is dosha specific.

Frequency for Kapha

Hearty, healthy Kapha is built sturdy with a lot of stamina. Kapha can have sex as often as desired, as long as they feel nourished. It's actually also good exercise for Kapha. Kapha is typically quite sensuous and easygoing with their curvy, full body, and soft belly. They are comfortable in their own skin and love to share, explore, and take their time. The other two doshas can benefit by learning these lessons from Kapha. They feel peaceful and blissful after sex, usually falling asleep with a smile on their lips.

Frequency for Vata

With less body weight and muscle mass, Vata doesn't have as much ojas as Kapha. Also, Vata can tend to feel anxious and nervous, and sexual stimulation can sometimes increase those emotions. Once a week may be all that Vata can handle. Vata needs to conserve energy, so take a look at how you are feeling. Perhaps cuddling and stroking may serve your needs. Vata can be scattered and unsure, so finding your voice and knowing what you need, and how to ask for it from your partner, is very important. There is nothing worse for Vata than doing something that goes against their wishes, as they will end up shaken, scared, confused, and might blame themselves. Vata can become cold and shaky after sex. It's important to stay warm and feel safe.

Frequency for Pitta

For Pitta, sex just a few times a month is best. Moderation is key as Pitta tends to go overboard with desires and urges. Pitta should be very aware of why they want to have sex. Since Pitta loves a challenge, they might be using sex to overcome inhibitions, show strength and dominance, or be unaware of their partner's true wishes. Listen, slow down, and be present with your partner. Do not have sex if you feel angry, frustrated, or impatient. Pitta may express anger or frustration during sex. Be on the lookout for this, and try to soften the experience by remembering that sex is an expression of love as well as an emotional release.

Dosha Partners

Two Kaphas together will naturally take their time and make long, slow love. They might consider spicing things up to burn a little bit more Kapha. Kapha will help Vata feel secure and safe, and can show Pitta a new level of sensitivity and sensuality. Two Vatas should be clear with each other about their level of stamina and scope of sexual actions. Two Pittas should be very aware of their feelings for each other, showing love and compassion—it's not a competition!

With regard to Pitta and Vata, more attention is needed. When Vata is balanced and feeling creative and spontaneous, they can guide Pitta into a healthy session of lovemaking. Playful Vata can help intense Pitta to lighten up a bit and enjoy sex without competition or power games. If Pitta is feeling balanced, they can take Vata by the hand as a leader and caretaker, gently offering guidance and helping Vata overcome fear and anxiety by being warm, kind, slow, and attentive. Beware, dear Vata: If your Pitta person is too intense, controlling, or angry, it is not the time for lovemaking, as this will make you anxious and fearful. Perhaps offer them a massage with a cooling oil such coconut oil, or a detox bath with Epsom salts and calming essential oils like lavender or vanilla.

Best Time of Day for Sex

Kapha time is usually the best time for sex. This is between 6 p.m. and 10 p.m. or between 6 a.m. and 10 a.m. The ideal time is 9 p.m. to 10 p.m. This is because Kapha time is slow, and one can take their time. And as with all physical and spiritual activity, it's best to have sex on an empty stomach, or at least two hours after eating. Ayurvedic texts advise you to avoid sex during the day, as daylight hours are to be used for other purposes.

Food Before and After Sex

It is advisable to have sex on an empty stomach; wait at least two to three hours after a meal. As mentioned earlier, sex depletes ojas, so you and your partner may want to share a concoction to rebuild your stamina. An ojas-rebuilding smoothie can be made with eight soaked and skinned almonds, three to six pitted dates, 16 ounces of warm almond milk, and a dash of nutmeg and cinnamon. Blend, and enjoy together. This is okay to drink before bed; in fact, it makes a nice evening drink, as its ingredients are calming.

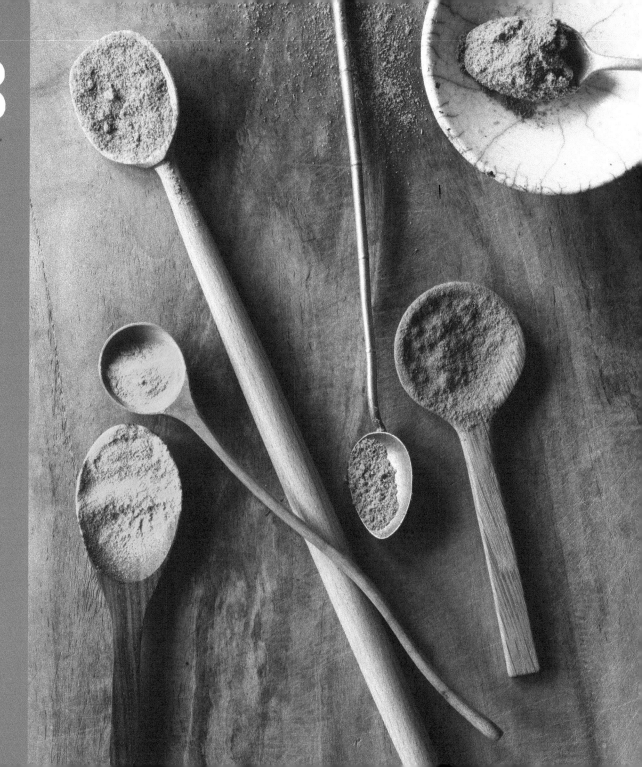

CHAPTER 8

Seasonal Adjustments and All-Season Cleanse

Knowing the seasons and their qualities, and making the appropriate adjustments, helps us be at our best. The ideal time to do an Ayurvedic cleanse to clear your body of toxins is at the change of seasons. In Ayurveda, we have three seasons, represented by all three doshas.

Vata season is late fall/early winter, typically November through February. The air turns colder, although some days are still warm. The atmosphere becomes drier, and leaves fall off the trees, but we still have heavy rains. It's changeable and unpredictable, just like Vata. Your skin becomes dry, and you may have some digestive issues, including gas and bloating, all representing too much Vata.

Kapha season is late winter/early spring, typically March through mid-June. The earth becomes heavy and saturated with snow and rain. We notice new growth occurring. The trees produce leaves again, and flowers and plants begin to poke their sprouts up from the ground. You might experience coughs, colds, and congestion as well as seasonal allergies, products of excess Kapha.

Pitta season is summer/early fall, typically mid-June through October. The heavy, cool rains of spring turn to humid, hot summer during Pitta season, along with angry thunderstorms. We tend to move more slowly through the heat, our appetite lessens, and the days become longer. Pitta season can show up quickly on your skin with rashes, sunburns, eczema, and other heat-related issues.

LATE FALL/EARLY WINTER (VATA) SEASONAL ADJUSTMENTS

The fall season begins when the leaves start falling from the trees, the rains lessen, and the air is cooler in the evening. As we move into late fall and early winter, the air becomes drier and we experience a mix of doshas—Pitta and Vata, soon settling into Vata for the duration until late winter.

This is Vata season. Just like the attributes of Vata, fall is changeable—hot one day, cold the next; rainy, then dry for a long spell. The winds come and dry the leaves as they fall to the ground. You may notice Vata qualities on the rise, even if your dosha is not primarily Vata. Skin becomes drier, behavior can become erratic, you may become constipated, and your hair and nails might feel brittle. During this season, it is important to reduce the tastes of bitter, pungent, and astringent and favor sweet, sour, and salty. These tastes/foods are naturally more densely nutritive and will add moisture and a feeling of groundedness to your body. This will help mitigate the effects of the season.

As we move deeper into the season, winter begins to feel like Mother Nature's permission to go within, quiet down, settle in, and nest a bit. By following the natural light of day, we begin to sleep in a little later and go to sleep a bit earlier.

Choose seasonal foods like root vegetables, and use warming spices like clove, cinnamon, and cayenne.

Late Fall/Early Winter Foods

Eat more sweet, sour, and salty. These are heavy, moist foods, such as soups and stews. Eat more protein in the winter months. Use ghee and warming spices such as cayenne, hot chiles, hing, nutmeg, and cinnamon.

Your shopping list should include avocados, beets, garlic, ginger, leeks, potatoes, pumpkin, root vegetables, winter squash, sweet fruits, ghee, avocado oil, sunflower oil, sesame seed oil, toasted sesame seed oil, eggs and fish, nuts and seeds, kefir, whole milk, cottage cheese, honey, maple syrup, molasses, Sucanat (whole cane sugar), tofu, mung beans, rice, quinoa, warming spices, warming teas (ginger, cinnamon, clove).

SUGGESTED DAILY ROUTINE

- Rise just after sunrise, perform your morning routine (see page 50), using sesame seed oil for oil pulling (see page 84).

- Use warm sesame seed oil or a Vata-reducing oil blend for your oil massage (see page 86). Oil the soles of your feet for extra grounding. Wipe your feet off before entering the shower. Leave a light sheen of oil on your skin to prevent it from drying and to protect it from environmental toxins.

- Use nasya oil in your nose and ears (see page 89). (Using a neti pot is not recommended in the dry season or in dry climates.)

- Use grounding and warming essential oils, such as vetiver, rose, and fir needle. (To use essential oils, see page 90.)

- Practice Alternate Nostril Breathing (see page 116).

- Perform slow, grounding yoga poses, such as Sun Salutation (page 102) and twists to move toxins out of the body.

- Eat warm, cooked foods. Avoid raw and cold foods. Use ghee in your cooking. Eat more soups and stews.

- Reduce foods that cause gas. To help with digestion, use a pinch of hing in your dishes. You can also chew roasted fennel seeds after meals.

- Drink hot/warm fluids throughout the day—ginger tea made with a few slices of raw ginger in hot water is ideal.

- The weather can be unpredictable (just like Vata), so dress in layers.

- Wear Vata-reducing (calming) colors: yellow, brown, beige, deep blue, indigo, gold, and burgundy.

- Perform your evening routine (see page 52).

- Drink Golden Milk (see page 60) before bed to help you sleep and reduce inflammation.

- Get into bed by around 9 p.m. or 10 p.m.

LATE WINTER/SPRING (KAPHA) SEASONAL ADJUSTMENTS

Typically, in most climates in springtime, the ground becomes heavy with rain, and the earth is abundant with new growth; flowers, bushes, and trees begin sprouting all around us. The heaviness and dampness of the earth translates to Kapha. Excess fluid creates Kapha. The budding of flora and fauna can cause allergies. The pressure of barometric changes can make us feel heavy and stagnant.

This season is Kapha—slow, heavy, wet, and cold. We will want to mitigate the Kaphic qualities in our food by reducing foods that are watery in nature—that is, those that fall into the sweet, sour, and salty categories. The wet atmosphere encourages us to eat lighter, drier foods. Since the air is often still cool, eat warm, cooked foods. Since the ground is heavy, eat foods that increase energy and motivation.

Late Fall/Spring Foods

Foods should be Kapha-reducing—more pungent, bitter, and astringent, which wring out excess fluid and toxins in the body. This time of year, you can eat brown rice, vegetable stews, and roasted foods. Avoid sweet, sour, and salty foods. Eliminate foods like ice cream, yogurt, hard cheeses, and heavy breads.

Your shopping list should include leafy greens, broccoli, celery, cauliflower, cabbage, dandelion greens, ginger, green beans, mushrooms, onions, potatoes, peas, watercress, apples, berries, dried fruits, pears, pomegranates, goat's milk, flaxseed oil, ghee, coconut oil, all spices, adzuki beans, urad dal, chickpeas, lentils, mung beans, eggs, seeds, amaranth, quinoa, millet, corn, buckwheat, rye, honey, maple syrup, Sucanat (whole cane sugar), alfalfa tea, clove tea, hibiscus tea, and cardamom tea.

SUGGESTED DAILY ROUTINE

- Rise with the sun, or just before, to get the Kapha moving and perform your morning routine (see page 50), using sesame seed oil for oil pulling (see page 84).

- Oil your body (see page 86), if you'd like, but consider dry brushing (see page 86) instead, if the oil causes you to feel heavy.

- Use nasya oil in your nose and ears (see page 89). If you live in a humid climate, use your neti pot (see page 88). Remember, do not use nasya oil until at least an hour after you use the neti pot, so you don't trap any water in your nasal passages or sinuses. Do not use the neti pot if you live in a dry climate, as it will further dry you out.

- Practice Bellows Breath to get excess Kapha out of your system (see page 118).

- Drink a glass of hot water with lemon or lime with 1 tablespoon of honey to "scrape" off Kapha, added only after the water cools off a bit.

- Use uplifting essential oils like clove, ginger, lemon, and jasmine. (To use essential oils, see page 90.)

- Increase the duration of your yoga poses. Practice chest openers, forward and back bends, and Sun Salutation (page 102).

- Get moderate to vigorous exercise several days a week.

- Wear a scarf around your throat to protect you from the shifting elements.

- Carry a Thermos with warm ginger water and sip it throughout the day.

- Wear Kapha-reducing colors: bright reds, oranges, greens, and blues.

- Perform your evening routine.

- Get into bed a little bit later than you do in the late fall/early winter, as the day grows longer.

SUMMER (PITTA) SEASONAL ADJUSTMENTS

Interestingly, during the summer our digestive "fires" (*agni*) are low. You might notice that you tend not to feel as hungry as you do in the winter. With more heat outside of our bodies, the internal agni is drawn out to the skin, and the interior of the body is cooled down, so we feel less hungry, but we still feel hotter on the outside. Therefore, you will notice an increase in skin issues in the summer like rashes, eczema, and other skin problems.

Summer Foods

Cool is the word for summer. Eat more sweet, bitter, and astringent foods. This is the time of year when you can eat salads and more fresh fruit (but not together). Avoid foods that add extra heat, such as spicy foods and hot drinks. Ice cream every once in a while is okay during the summer, because it contains "vitamin H"— *vitamin happy*!

Your shopping list should include asparagus, avocados, beet greens, bitter melon, broccoli, corn, cucumbers, coconuts, jicama, kale, parsley, cilantro, watercress, zucchini, apples, apricots, berries, melons, sweet cherries, dried fruit, sweet citrus, pineapples, pomegranates, eggs, adzuki beans, chickpeas, lentils, mung beans, tofu, almond oil, avocado oil, coconut oil, ghee, fennel, peppermint, spearmint, barley, rice, rye, wheat, dandelion tea, mint tea, stinging nettle tea, maple syrup, Sucanat (whole cane sugar), almonds, pine nuts, seeds, whole milk, and kefir.

SUGGESTED DAILY ROUTINE

- Rise before sunrise, while it's still cool, and perform your morning routine (see page 50).

- Use a drop or two of peppermint or spearmint essential oil on your toothbrush before brushing.

- Oil your body (see page 86), using coconut oil.

- Use cooling essential oils such as sandalwood, floral scents (such as jasmine), and sweet scents (such as citrus, lemon, or lime). Fill a spritzer with distilled water and add 10 to 15 drops of your favorite oil, and carry

it with you to cool down as needed.
(To use essential oils, see page 90.)

- Use nasya oil in your nose and ears (see page 89). If you live in a humid climate, use your neti pot (see page 88). Remember, do not use nasya oil until at least an hour after you use the neti pot so you don't trap any water in your nasal passages or sinuses. Do not use the neti pot if you live in a dry climate, as it will further dry you out.

- Practice Cooling Breath as needed (see page 117).

- Stay hydrated with cool, but not chilled, drinks. Try mint tea, Everyday CCF Tea (see page 57), fennel tea, coconut water, or cucumber water.

- Eat an easy-to-digest dinner.

- Dress in pure cotton or linen. White feels cooler, but the rays of the sun can still penetrate the material. Use a natural sunscreen. You can make your own (see page 151), but be sure to get adequate sun in the morning and early evening without sunblock to boost your body's production of vitamin D. Sun gazing is a good way to do this (see page 124).

- Conserve your energy and avoid overheating by reducing vigorous exercise. Perform gentle yoga poses, such as chest openers, gentle stretches, and twists.

- Wear Pitta-reducing colors: cooling light blues and greens, white, tan, cool gray, pastel colors, pink, and soft rose.

- Perform your evening routine.

- Get into bed around 10 p.m. or 11 p.m. Resist the urge to be a night owl in the summer.

ALL-SEASON CLEANSE

What makes this cleanse seasonal is that it is performed at the change of seasons, so ideally, you would be doing this three times a year, or as needed. When first getting familiar with a cleanse, take it slow and listen to your body. Here are a few guidelines and tips to keep in mind:

- Make sure you have three to five days to do the cleanse. It is best not to be working or involved in anything stressful during this period.

- Have all your cooking ingredients handy so you won't have to go searching around for that elusive spice, grain, or bean.

- Avoid a cleanse during your menstrual cycle or if pregnant.

- Have the following personal items handy: tongue scraper, dry brush, oil for body massage, and triphala tablets or powder.

- All doshas will notice changes in mood, energy level, hunger, and comfort or discomfort during a cleanse. Since this is a detox, you might notice that you feel tired, crampy, or achy—but it will pass. You should be cleansed and begin to feel rejuvenated by midway through the process.

- All doshas should do a body oil massage or dry brush every morning to get the lymph system moving.

- Breath work is key. Practice Alternate Nostril Breathing (see page 116) every day for at least 5 minutes—preferably in the morning, but anytime is good.

- Avoid excessive exercise. Just do some easy walking during Kapha time of day—between either 6 a.m. and 10 a.m. or 6 p.m. and 10 p.m. You can also take a 10-minute walk after your meals to aid digestion.

- Avoid cold drinks. Sip Everyday CCF Tea (see page 57) or just plain warm or hot water with a few slices of gingerroot throughout the day.

- Avoid coffee, tobacco and related products, recreational drugs, and alcohol. The only things you should be taking into your body during your cleanse are listed here.

Performing the Cleanse

For this cleanse, you will follow a modified kitchari mono-diet. For Pitta and Kapha, it is okay to do a juice fast for a few days in place of the kitchari mono-diet. Vata, however, should not do a liquid fast. Read all of the instructions carefully. All meal sizes are two handfuls of food, which represents 80 percent of your stomach—or two-thirds leaving 20 percent or one-third—open for your digestive "fires" to process the food.

DAYS 1 TO 3

1. Eat breakfast between 7 a.m. and 9 a.m.

Vata choices: citrus fruit and sweet seasonal fruit (e.g., berries, cherries, peaches, nectarines, and apricots). Avoid bananas. Alternatively, you can make a plain yogurt drink (*lassi*) with 2 cups of water, ½ cup of organic plain whole-fat yogurt, and 1 tablespoon of Sucanat (whole cane sugar).

Pitta choices: sweet fruits and berries, sweet grapes, peaches, nectarines.

Kapha choices: berries, sour fruit or slightly ripened fruit, cranberries, apples, grapes, apricots, pomegranates.

2. Eat lunch four hours after breakfast, between 11 a.m. and 1 p.m.

All doshas: Two handfuls of freshly made kitchari (see chapter 5 for your dosha's kitchari recipe). However, you can have a little more if you are really hungry.

3. Eat dinner four hours after lunch, but three hours before bed (between 4 p.m. and 6 p.m.). This is your lightest meal of the day:

All doshas: steamed vegetables or vegetable soup (not tomato-based)—just a simple broth with some vegetables. If you feel like you need it, perhaps add 1 handful of kitchari.

4. Before bed, wash your feet and oil them. Then do the following:

Pitta and Kapha: Take 3 triphala tablets.

Vata: In small pot, mix together 6 ounces of whole milk (or almond milk, if vegan) and 1 teaspoon of ghee or almond oil (if vegan). Bring it to a boil over medium heat. Allow it to cool down, and drink before bed. Take 2 triphala tablets.

DAYS 4 AND 5

Begin a castor oil–orange juice cleanse on day 4. Try to schedule this for when you can stay home and rest. Castor oil is a purgative, so stay close to a bathroom. Don't do any strenuous activities on this day. Try to rest, read, and take it easy.

1. Do not eat anything in the morning, keeping your stomach empty.

2. In a small glass, whisk together 1 teaspoon of castor oil with 4 to 6 ounces of orange juice. In place of the orange juice, you can eat an orange.

3. Drink the mixture or take the castor oil by spoon and eat the orange.

Vata: Wait until you feel hungry to eat something, and it should be only kitchari or vegetable soup. (Vata should not do a liquid fast.)

All doshas: Drink Everyday CCF Tea (page 57) throughout the day.

Pitta: After the castor oil–orange juice cleanse, do a lime water fast for one day. Mix a few teaspoons of lime juice into a pot of warm water and sip throughout the day.

Kapha: After the castor oil–orange juice cleanse, do a pomegranate juice fast for one day. Let the juice come to room temperature. Sip it throughout the day. You can alternate with lemon water and honey, if you'd like. You can use store-bought pomegranate juice or make it yourself from fresh produce.

TIP: If you did not have a good bowel movement on day 4, you can increase the castor oil to 1½ teaspoons to 1 tablespoon on day 5.

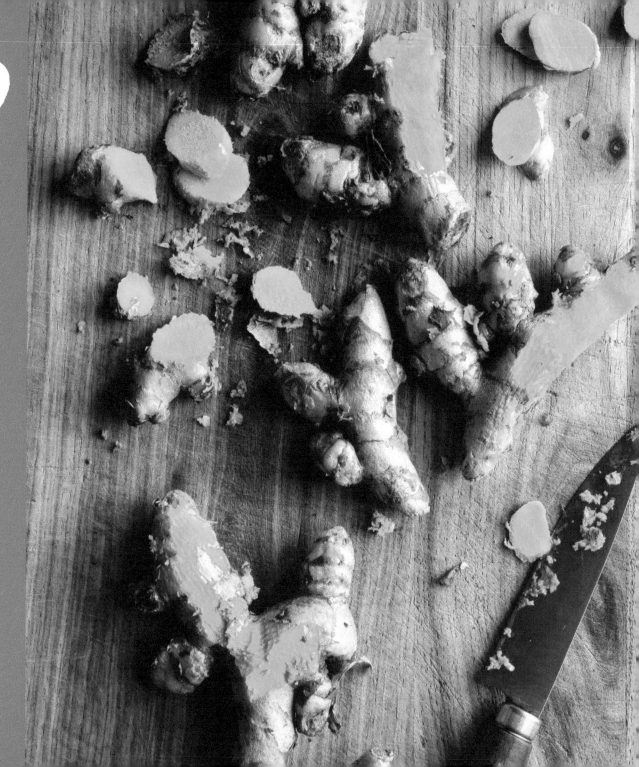

CHAPTER 9

Medicinal Herbs
and Remedies
for Common Ailments

Ayurveda is one of the best-known healing systems for disease prevention and longevity. The suggestions here for healing some common ailments should not be used as a substitute for medical attention. But if you do try these suggestions, you might find that your need for medical intervention will be less.

If you can catch your symptoms just as they begin—a tickle in the throat, a nagging ache in the back—you can heal them quickly with food, teas, essential oils, breath work, and movement. There is, though, knowledge to be gained in illness. It can be a good opportunity to go within and examine your life. Your body is trying to tell you something, so take this time to listen—and to fix it.

Let's first look at some healing herbal supplements that you may find fit the bill for helping reduce your particular symptoms. Some of these herbs may be ingredients you find in a recipe, but here we are specifically talking about supplements.

TOP AYURVEDIC MEDICINAL HERBS

An Ayurvedic practitioner may prescribe certain medicinal herbs to help relieve whatever is causing trouble; herbs may also be suggested as a daily supplement. You might find some or all of the following at your local health food store, but they are readily available for purchase over the Internet.

Choose products only from reputable companies, and be sure to read the product descriptions, common uses, and possible contraindications. If you are in any doubt, check with a practitioner before taking supplements. Avoid them if you are pregnant, unless you are told otherwise by your practitioner. Always tell your physician if you are taking any supplements.

1. **Ashwagandha**—adaptogenic; stress reducing; sleep aid by deeply relaxing nervous system—same function for reducing stress; energy; rest when you need it; joint support

2. **Bacopa**—brain booster; detox for blood and brain; calms the mind; aids in memory, concentration, and focus

3. **Boswellia (Indian frankincense)**—Ayurvedic "aspirin"; pain relief; joint support; reduces inflammation; balances blood sugar; promotes healthy complexion

4. **Ginger**—digestive aid; antioxidant; reduces inflammation; reduces toxins; helps settle the stomach post-meals and during travel

5. **Gymnema**—greatly reduces desire and craving for sugar and regulates appetite

6. **Neem**—promotes healthy teeth and skin; detoxes blood and liver

7. **Shatavari**—translates to "100 husbands" (as in a woman who takes this could service 100 husbands . . . if she is so inclined). Enhances libido; nourishes and supports a healthy female reproductive system at any age (equally important during the fertile years all the way through peri- and postmenopause); can help with breast milk production; supports digestion; helps the male reproductive system

8. **Triphala**—bowel toner; comprises three Ayurvedic super fruits: Amalaki, Bibhitaki, and Haritaki; lubricates the colon so that you can more efficiently absorb nutrients and more completely empty the bowels; antioxidant

9. **Tulsi (holy basil)**—all-over stress reducer; blood-sugar balancing; helps relieve pain; promotes mental clarity; promotes circulation

10. **Turmeric**—anti-inflammatory; joint support; digestive aid; brain booster

COMMON AILMENTS

Everyone would like to avoid a trip to the doctor when they can, but *always* seek the advice of a professional if your symptoms are particularly bad, or if they persist or get worse despite your best efforts to care for yourself. The remedies in this section may ease your symptoms, as they do for the many, so do give them a try.

Arthritis

- Steep a cup of ginger tea by heating water and adding a few slices of fresh ginger. Add a tablespoon of castor oil. Drink before going to bed.

- Use sesame seed oil or mahanarayan oil (see the resources on page 161) to oil your joints morning and night. Use about a teaspoon of oil, and massage it on to your problem joints.

Constipation

- Add a tablespoon of psyllium powder (available at health food stores or online) to an 8-ounce glass of water, and drink it in the morning and evening. You can also add psyllium to food or soup.

- Take 2 to 3 triphala tablets before bed with warm water.

- Take 2 tablespoons of aloe vera gel mixed with water or juice once a day. Or drink 8 ounces of aloe vera juice, once or twice a day depending on the severity of the symptom. If you are pregnant, speak to your practitioner before using aloe vera.

- Boil 6 ounces of whole cow's milk or goat's milk (or nondairy milk if you are vegan). Stir in 1 teaspoon of ghee (use almond oil if vegan). Drink before bed every night for at least seven days. You should have immediate relief. After a week, use as needed.

- Rub your belly with warm castor oil before going to sleep.

Cough and Cold

- Make a steam inhalation using 3 drops of lavender essential oil, 3 drops of eucalyptus essential oil, and 3 drops of tea tree oil in a pot of hot water. Place a towel over your head, lean over the bowl, and inhale deeply, alternating between breathing through the nose and mouth, for five minutes. Take a break, and do it again for another five minutes. Do this twice a day.

- Use a neti pot if you have a runny nose. Do not use a neti pot if your nasal passages are clogged, but you can use nasya oil as needed. Remember to *never* use nasya oil in the nose right after using your neti pot.

Doing so can trap water in the nasal passages, leading to infection. Wait at least one hour between these practices.

- Mix equal parts raw organic honey with organic cinnamon. One tablespoon of each should suffice. Add a drop or two of warm water to make a paste. Lick it off a spoon. It will knock your socks off and knock your cold out!

- Drink licorice tea if you have a cough. There are many brands on the market, including Breathe Deep Yogi Tea. It helps open the lungs and reduces phlegm.

Cough, Dry

- Make a steam inhalation using 3 to 5 drops of eucalyptus oil in a pot of hot water. Place a towel over your head, lean over the bowl, and inhale deeply, alternating between breathing through the nose and mouth, for 5 minutes. Take a break, and do it again for another 5 minutes. Do this two or three times a day.

- Gargle with ½ teaspoon of salt and ½ teaspoon of turmeric powder in warm water.

- Drink hot tea made with a pinch each of ginger powder, ground cardamom, and ground cinnamon.

- Drink licorice tea, to which you have added 10 drops of mahanarayan oil. Sip the tea throughout the day.

Cough, Wet

- For a wet cough, try the Ayurvedic herbal powders sitopaladi or talisadi (and mixed with 1 tablespoon of raw organic honey for an added boost, if desired).

- Steep a cup of ginger tea by heating water and adding a few slices of fresh ginger. Drink throughout the day. Add 1 tablespoon of raw organic honey, if desired.

- Drink licorice tea throughout the day. Add 1 tablespoon of raw organic honey, if desired.

Diarrhea

- Make a cup of lassi with ½ cup of warm water and ½ cup of plain, whole-fat organic yogurt and a pinch of salt. Drink it down.

- Drink Everyday CCF Tea (page 57) throughout the day.

- Eat one very ripe banana each day until the diarrhea passes; do not eat the banana with other food.

- Avoid hot, spicy food.

- Make boiled rice (*kanji*) by bring 6 to 8 cups of water to a boil; add 1 cup brown or white basmati rice; add ½ teaspoon turmeric powder, ½ teaspoon ginger powder, and a pinch of salt. Let the mixture simmer, covered, for an hour. Eat the rice and drink the leftover water.

Dry Eyes

A technique called *netra basti*, a treatment for the eyes, can be self-administered, but if you have any doubt about doing it, speak to an Ayurvedic practitioner. To do this, follow these instructions:

1. Warm up a few tablespoons of ghee. Using clean swimming goggles, fill each goggle with the warm (not hot!) ghee.

2. Bend over a sink or bowl, and place the goggles on your eyes. Place the head strap in place and lie down on the floor or bed with a towel under you to catch any ghee that escapes. (Keep the bowl by your side for when you remove the goggles.)

3. Keep your eyes open and move your eyeballs around in a circular motion. Stay like this for 10 to 20 minutes. Close your eyes if rest is needed, but the idea is to slowly move your eyes around the whole time.

4. Turn to the side and bend over the bowl to remove the goggles. Wipe your eyes with a clean cotton cloth and rest with your eyes closed for 10 minutes.

5. Repeat several times a week until the problem disappears.

Ear Infections

I've heard that babies in India rarely get ear infections, and that can probably be attributed to the practice of ear oiling (*karna purana*). It's also a remedy for tinnitus and chronic ear infections. Other benefits include relief from age-related hearing loss and detoxification of the ear canal. It's also very relaxing. To perform ear oiling:

1. Using sesame seed oil or nasya oil, warm a small bottle in hot water and test on your skin before using.

2. Using a dropper, tilt your head to one side and fill your ear with 6 to 10 drops of oil. It can be a strange sensation and might send shivers down your spine, but you will soon relax into it.

3. Using your index finger and middle finger, massage the area around your ears, the cartilage, and behind your ear. Close the ear flap for a few seconds, and pull your ear lobe down a few times; then lie down for about 10 minutes.

4. Before oiling the other side, place a cotton ball in your ear to catch any leftover oil. Alternatively, you can lie down and have someone place the drops in your ear for you.

Gas

- Avoid raw foods.

- Chew on roasted fennel seeds after a meal.

- Cook foods with digestive spices such as cumin, hing, ajwain seeds, and ginger.

- Remember, in Ayurveda, we don't suppress urges, so if you have gas, just let it pass.

Headache

- See the entry for "pain."

- Make sure you are well hydrated, completely avoiding cold drinks and food.

- Breathe deeply, do Alternate Nostril Breathing (see page 116) several times a day.

- Massage your head, scalp, and neck with seasonal oil.

- Boswellia is a great pain reliever.

Heartburn

- For heartburn, do Cooling Breath (see page 117) to cool down your body.

- Take 1 tablespoon of aloe vera juice mixed with ¼ teaspoon of baking soda.

- Take 2 tablespoons of apple cider vinegar in 6 ounces of warm water.

- Drink omam water (see the entry for "pain" for instructions to make this water).

- See the remedies for indigestion as well.

Indigestion

- Avoid overeating, and eat at least three hours before bed.

- Don't snack between meals.

- Don't mix fruit and other foods.

- Lie on your left side to encourage digestion by supporting your stomach.

- Avoid spicy foods and raw foods.

- Drink warm water with lime.

Irritable Bowels

- Eat only cooked foods, and avoid all raw food. Also avoid milk, sweets, caffeine, alcohol, and nightshade vegetables.

- Use light oils like sunflower and safflower.

- Take probiotics or eat probiotic foods such as chickpeas, asparagus, apples, lentils, and pomegranates.

- Take easy walks, especially after eating.

Lack of Hunger

- Don't snack between meals.

- Spark your digestive "fires" by eating a small slice of ginger with a sprinkle of salt about 30 minutes before a meal.

- Drink a small glass of warm water 30 minutes before a meal.

Low Libido/Vaginal Dryness

- Women with a low libido can take the herbal supplement shatavari. This herbal medicinal supplement helps with mental stimulation, as well as combatting vaginal dryness. You can use coconut oil topically if dryness persists.

- Men with low libido can take the herbal supplement ashwagandha (meaning "strength of a horse"). This herb is so nourishing in general, but in this context, it can help calm the nervous system and direct attention toward the task at hand.

- Ashwagandha is a known as an aphrodisiac that can help both men and women get in the mood.

Menopause

- Each dosha may experience menopause differently: Vata may display depression, anxiety, insomnia, and general fatigue. Pitta may suffer from hot flashes, headaches, and bouts of anger and rage. Kapha may gain weight, feel tired and foggy, and have low energy. See an Ayurvedic practitioner for individualized treatment.

- Increase consumption of phytoestrogenic foods (must be organic and non-GMO), including sweet potatoes, flaxseeds, oat bran, barley bran, miso, tempeh, dried dates, tofu, cashews, hazelnuts, broccoli, and mung beans.

- Take the medicinal herb shatavari to help keep the reproductive tissues lubricated and robust.

- Consider the herbal remedy vidari kanda powder, which supports the reproductive tissues and strengthens muscles and nerves.

- Lime juice and pomegranate juice have been reported to relieve hot flashes and other symptoms.

- To relieve hot flashes, use Cooling Breath (see page 117) to cool down the system, especially during a hot flash. Practice Alternate Nostril Breathing (see page 116) every day for 15 minutes.

Menstrual Cramps

- Medicinal herbs like shatavari, aswaghandha, and tulsi can help regulate, detox, and reduce pain connected to menstruation.

- Triphala tablets can be helpful.

- Performing dry brushing and body oil massage (*abhyanga*) helps remove stagnation and toxins from the body.

- Eat a simple diet, drink plenty of warm fluids, and avoid raw foods.

Muscle Aches

- Apply mahanarayan oil and Tiger Balm liniment liberally to the areas involved, and massage deeply after a hot shower.

- Take herbs for pain relief and anti-inflammatory properties, including Boswellia, guggulu, and ashwagandha.

Nausea

- Cooling peppermint tea and cooling, minty essential oils like peppermint and spearmint can help reduce nausea.

- Nibbling ginger in many forms, such as raw ginger or crystalized ginger, can relieve nausea caused by traveling or driving.

- Be sure not to eat foods that don't digest well together, such as raw fruit with any other food.

Pain

- Ajwain seeds can be used similarly to aspirin, as it contains a pain-relieving chemical called thymol. To make a pain reliever called omam water, steep a teaspoon of ajwain seeds in 10 ounces of hot water for at least 10 minutes, or overnight. Sip for relief. Scientific research has found 24 medicinally active compounds in each seed. Ajwain seeds are used as an all-purpose healer for many ailments, including asthma, coughs and colds, pain relief, and infection-causing bacteria.

- Omam water is also beneficial as an antacid for heartburn, as a pain reliever for headaches, and as an antihistamine for allergies.

Seasonal Allergies

- Omam water acts as an antihistamine. (See the "pain" entry to prepare this water.)

- Kapha often suffer from upper respiratory ailments, especially in spring.

- Take a tablespoon of raw organic honey every day during allergy season.

- Use a neti pot every day, and follow up with nasya oil about an hour later.

- The Ayurvedic herb trikatu can help clear out excess Kapha.

- Use a dry brush to stimulate the lymph system and help get rid of toxins.

- Make sure to include plenty of pungent and bitter herbs, spices, and foods in your diet, including leafy greens, cayenne pepper, basil, ginger, and cardamom (for Kapha).

- Pitta displays seasonal allergies in spring and summer, usually with itchy, burning eyes, rashes, inflammation, and headaches.

- Use Ayurvedic herbs to calm and cool the body including neem, Amalaki, and Guduchi (for Pitta).

- Use a Pitta-cooling oil for oiling the body (for Pitta).

- Avoid spicy food, and add lots of coriander, fennel, cilantro, and coconut to your food.

- Drink cool (not chilled) coconut water (for Pitta).

- Dandelion tea and stinging nettle tea can be sipped throughout the day (for Pitta).

- Vata usually feels seasonal allergies in the fall. They can come down with dry, itchy eyes, a sore throat and dry cough, and sometimes even generalized fatigue, muscle aches, and soreness.

- A warm Epsom salt bath will do wonders for Vata.

- Add extra ghee to the diet (for Vata).

- Take the herb ashwagandha to boost the immune system and calm allergens (for Vata).

- Make sure to drink plenty of hot tea—ginger with lemon is great; add a big scoop of honey after the tea has cooled off slightly (for Vata and Kapha).

- Use a Vata-calming oil for oiling the body (for Vata).

Stress and Anxiety

- Practice meditation daily.

- Listen to chants or spiritual music.

- Go on a media "fast"—no TV, radio, newspaper, or Internet.

- Include good oils in your diet like ghee, avocado, and olive.

- Try stress-reducing herbs like aswaghandha, jatamansi, licorice, and calamus root.

- Reduce your intake of caffeine (unless that causes you further stress. If so, reduce gradually).

- Use calming essential oils like lavender, vanilla, and sandalwood.

- Practice Cobra Pose (see page 103), Cat and Cow Poses (see page 97), and Sun Salutation (see page 102).

Sunburn

- Rub aloe gel liberally onto the sunburned skin. If you have access to an aloe vera plant, then cut open one of its leaves and use the gel directly from the plant.

- Mix equal amounts of powdered sandalwood and turmeric with a little cool water and apply the paste directly to the sunburn.

- Apply pads of cold, strong, black tea directly to the sunburned skin with soaked cotton pads several times a day.

Natural Sunscreen Recipe

¼ cup avocado, almond, or olive oil

½ cup coconut oil

3 to 5 drops each citronella, lemongrass, and geranium essential oils (mosquito repellant; optional)

2 to 4 tablespoons non-nano micronized zinc oxide

1. Combine the oils and the mosquito repellent, if using, in a small to medium glass jar, such as a mason jar.

2. In a saucepan, heat a small amount of water until warm, and place the opened jar in the water to melt the coconut oil.

3. When the oil melts, remove the jar from the water, put the lid on, and shake to mix.

4. Open the jar and add the zinc oxide, being careful not to inhale the particles. Stir it in.

Et voilà! Sunscreen. Store at room temperature or in the fridge. It will become solid. This is not waterproof, so reapply it often while outdoors.

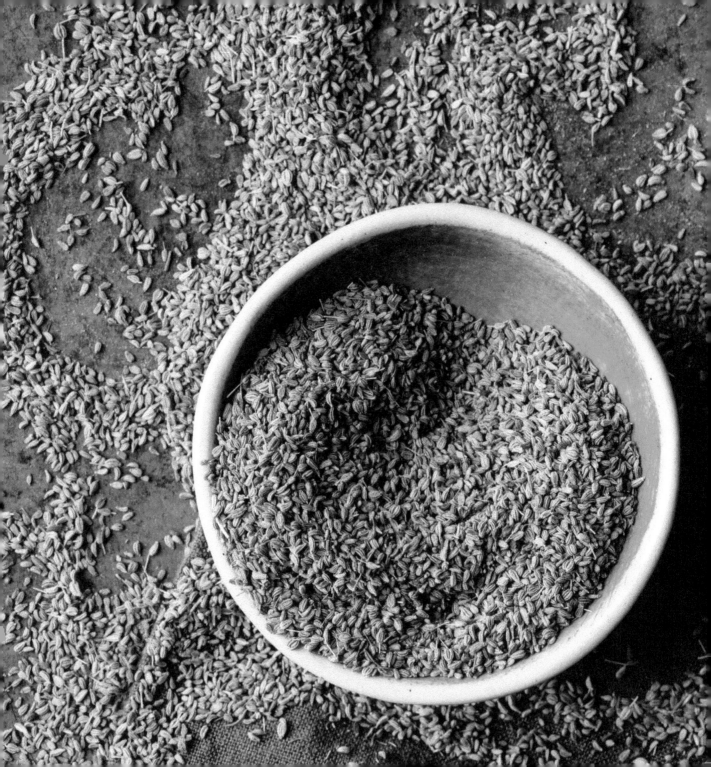

COMMON AYURVEDIC COOKING INGREDIENTS

Ajwain seeds (bishop's weed)—This is a potent, flavorful spice that tastes like celery seed, thyme, and anise. Its flavor mellows with cooking. There is no need to grind the seeds; they soften as they cook. If you add them just before serving, they are slightly crunchy. Use celery seed if you can't find this spice. You may also see it spelled *ajowan* or *ajman*.

Avocado oil—This high-heat oil is rich in vitamin E and omega-3 fatty acids. It is undeniably healthy, but a little on the expensive side. Avocado oil's smooth flavor adds another dimension to your cooking. Do not refrigerate it. It is best for Vata and Pitta, and Kapha should use it moderately.

Black mustard seeds—This flavorful, but tiny, seed contains many health-promoting properties. In cooking, they are like the canary in the coal mine—they let you know when the oil is just the right temperature for adding the other ingredients: They pop just as they hit the right temperature.

Bragg's Liquid Aminos—This soy product is a super-flavorful alternative to soy and tamari sauce. It does not contain table salt or any preservatives or dyes, but it does contain essential amino acids.

Chia seeds—This superfood is a fabulous source of omega-3 fatty acids. It's great to use in vegan muffins or brownies and other recipes because the seeds plump up and retain moisture.

Cilantro—These are the leaves of the coriander plant. Cilantro is fantastic for detoxing. It's great for juicing, and using in soups and as a garnish.

Cinnamon (ground)—This delicious spice is known to balance blood sugar and may be helpful in preventing diabetes. It's both sweet and spicy at the same time. The recipes in chapter 5 call for ground cinnamon, but you can get creative with whole cinnamon sticks and add one to your soups and stews while cooking.

Clove buds and ground cloves—Cloves are an ancient remedy for toothaches, and for healthy gums and teeth. The oil of the clove is an anesthetic. It can boost circulation and reduce inflammation, thus promoting healing. It's also antibacterial—an amazing healing package in a little bud. Remove whole cloves from a dish before serving. A few whole cloves, as well as ground cloves go a long way.

Coriander seeds and ground coriander—The seeds are great in steeping teas, or whole in soups and stews. Ground coriander adds a lovely flavor to dishes. The health benefits include digestive aid, easing constipation, decreasing bad cholesterol, and increasing good cholesterol. Mixing whole seeds with your black peppercorns in a grinder makes for a delightful addition to salads, soups, and stews.

Cumin seeds and ground cumin—Cumin's main compound is *cuminaldehyde*; it is a super-antioxidant that contains medicinal qualities, such as combatting diabetes, reducing blood pressure, and building stronger bones.

Curry leaves—Medicinally, curry leaves are used in India to treat everything from infections and inflammation to controlling diabetes and heart disease. You can eat them, or remove them after cooking. If you can't find them, leave them out, because there is just no substitute. But do try to find them, as the flavor is unbeatable! They freeze well, so if you can get them, purchase extra for another time.

Daikon radish—The health benefits of this milder radish are vast. They help clear out your respiratory tract, promote digestive health, aid in detoxification, bolster your immunity, and alleviate inflammation. I could go on about this amazing radish, but I think you get the idea.

Dried chickpeas—You'll find these little power-houses, also called garbanzo beans, in the dried bean section of your grocery store. Make an effort to buy only organic or otherwise this crop is heavily sprayed with pesticides. If you purchase canned chickpeas instead, also be sure to buy organic.

Fennel seed—Fennel is a licorice-like herb and a spice. Full of phytoestrogens, the seeds can work wonders for menopausal women and can relieve menstrual cramps. It is also known to be anti-inflammatory, making this a natural Pitta-reducing spice. It's also known for easing digestion.

Flaxseeds—Keep whole flaxseeds on hand, and store them in the refrigerator, as they can become rancid quickly. Grind them as needed for your recipes. I suggest not purchasing ground flaxseed, as it begins to lose its potency as soon as the seeds are ground. They are a fantastic source of omega-3 fatty acids, and the slightly nutty flavor is delicious. Do not heat. Flaxseeds are to be added to food after it is cooked, used in salad dressings, or added to juices.

Ginger (fresh) and ginger powder—The root of the ginger plant, whether fresh or dried and powdered, has an amazing array of healing qualities, and should be a staple in any kitchen—Ayurvedic or otherwise. Gingerroot powder is best for Kapha, and raw ginger is better for Vata and Pitta, because it is moist.

Hing (asafetida)—This is a resin from the fennel plant. It is an essential cooking ingredient that helps you digest your beans and other foods that may cause gas. It is most balancing for Vata and has good heating qualities for Kapha. Use it sparingly for Pitta. It has a very strong smell that becomes milder when cooked. I store mine in a plastic bag in the freezer to keep my kitchen from smelling like it (some say the smell is akin to dirty socks). A pinch is all you need in most dishes.

Honey—Always purchase raw organic honey. The processing of conventional honey kills the many beneficial qualities of this sweet and nutritious gift from the bees. *Never* heat honey.

Jaggery—Jaggery is the name for Indian boiled sugarcane solids. It's a form of lightly processed sugar that is super sweet and yummy. It comes in a block or cone of brown, soft jaggery. You can find this at an Indian store or a great organic brand from Pure Indian Foods at www.pureindianfoods.com. It also comes in a powdered form.

Kombu—This seaweed, which comes in dried strips, is an excellent seasoning in soups and for adding powerful sea minerals to your food. The kombu can be eaten or removed after cooking. One piece adds a powerful punch.

Miso—Miso is made from fermented soybeans. White miso is fermented soybeans with a large percentage of rice. It's mild and sweet. Yellow miso is usually made from soybeans that have been fermented with barley. This miso has a mild, earthy flavor. Red miso is also made with soybeans fermented with barley and other grains, with more soybeans and a longer fermentation time. It has a heavier flavor than the mild, yellow version. You can use any color you want, and you may even find some new kinds in the market, as fermented foods are gaining in popularity. Experiment with them to see which flavor you like best. In hearty soups and stews, you may like red. If making a salad dressing, white or yellow is the best way to go so as not to overpower the flavor of the veggies.

Mung beans—You should be able to easily find dried, whole mung beans (also called dal), which are green. Split yellow mung beans are a little harder to find; they are the whole green mung bean that has been processed to split open. The green hull falls off and leaves the yellow insides, making it easier for cooking and easier to absorb the nutrients. Mung beans are a common ingredient in Ayurvedic dishes, so try to keep them as staples in your kitchen. All Indian stores will carry these two staples.

Nutmeg (ground)—You can buy whole nutmeg and grind it as needed (a microplaner works great) for the freshest version. If you buy already ground nutmeg, be sure to keep the jar sealed tight to prevent losing the essential oils that make this powerful spice so special.

Olive oil—If you enjoy cooking, you likely already have this oil in your kitchen, but for your Ayurvedic kitchen, choose organic extra-virgin olive oil. Others olive oils may contain a blend of oils. Compared to other oils, this can go bad relatively fast. Be sure to keep it sealed and in a cool dark place. Olive oil usually comes in a dark glass container or a tin for this purpose. You don't want to expose it to bright light.

Pea protein powder—Unlike protein powders made from whey, pea protein powder is entirely vegan, and it packs a protein punch.

Pumpkin seeds—It's best to buy raw, unsalted seeds. They are a great source of zinc. To really make them pop, so to speak, toss a handful into a hot saucepan and heat until they begin to pop. Remove immediately and add to soups, vegetables, or just eat them on their own.

Quinoa—Grown in the Andes, this is actually a seed, not a grain. As a seed, it contains protein, so it's a great choice for vegetarians and vegans. Just be sure to wash it, as it's coated with a naturally occurring phytochemical called saponin. The bitter-tasting saponin protects the plant from pests. In addition to washing the quinoa well to remove the saponin, you can soak the seeds in water overnight, which will sprout them a bit. Rinse again and cook. It will be even more nutritious.

Red lentils—Also called masoor dal in Indian food stores, this lentil actually turns yellow when cooked. It's very nutritious and hearty. I like to soak them before cooking while I prep the other ingredients. As with all beans and lentils, this is a great source of easily digestible protein, will reduce cholesterol, and is heart healthy.

Sunflower oil—Make sure to buy unrefined, organic oil to preserve all the healthy benefits of this light-tasting oil. Sunflower seeds are full of antioxidants, like vitamin E and tocopherols, so even though this oil is high in omega-6 fatty acids (omega-3s are healthier), it's still a relatively good oil, especially for high-heat cooking.

Tofu—Tofu is made from soybean curd and is best eaten in moderation by all three doshas (and very limited for Kapha, as it's heavy and cold). It's extremely important to buy only organic, as the nonorganic versions are all genetically modified. Soft or silken tofu is great for making vegan desserts. It blends up like cream.

Turmeric powder (*Curcuma longa*)—This yellow-colored spice, which is related to ginger, is a star in Indian cooking. It has a long list of health benefits due to many bioactive compounds called curcuminoids, including anti-inflammatory and antioxidant properties. Be sure to purchase only organic turmeric, as nonorganic may contain heavy metals from the soil. You can also buy the root, called a rhizome, and grate it yourself for use in cooking. You may find that your fingers and cutting board are stained yellow, but don't worry, it washes off easily.

White basmati rice—White basmati rice is easier to digest than brown rice. It's a mainstay of the Ayurvedic diet, so don't be scared of this healthy carbohydrate. Basmati rice contains thiamin and niacin, two B vitamins, as well as vitamins E and K and magnesium. With a low-glycemic level, it's good for people with diabetes. It also has more fiber than other white rice.

THE THREE UNIVERSAL QUALITIES AND THE FIVE SHEATHS

THREE UNIVERSAL QUALITIES (GUNAS)

There are three subtle qualities found in nature, each of which is related to a dosha. They are *sattva*, *rajas*, and *tamas*.

- **Sattva** (Vata): Pure, calm, alert, sweet. Sattva is the observer. Sattva is the ability to see and perceive goodness in the world and in yourself. There is a sweetness, calmness, and contentedness in life.

- **Rajas** (Pitta): Momentum, aggravation, activity. Rajas is the observation. Rajas comes in and stirs things up, questions, and moves things around.

- **Tamas** (Kapha): Inactive, dull, heavy. Tamas is the object being observed. Tamas slows things down, lacks awareness, creates inaction, and confusion.

These universal qualities literally bind us to nature through our energetic body as well as through our physical body, our karma, and our consciousness.

THE FIVE SHEATHS (KOSHAS)

The word *kosha* literally means "covering" or "sheath." In healing ourselves, we are able to break free of the koshas that bind us in our thinking, our bodies, and our beliefs—we can move through the koshas and embrace the cosmic truth in the center of our being: that there is no separation between us and every other being on earth.

We are all part of an interconnected web, and every action we take affects everything else. Think of the ocean. The body of water and waves that rise up and then lap the shore are all made of tiny drops, but the entire ocean could not exist without each drop. Our world could not exist without you and your personal contribution to the whole—just as the ocean could not exist without the drops that comprise it.

The koshas are literally layer upon layer of consciousness that wraps around our existence, like lampshade upon lampshade, with a lightbulb of pure consciousness shining in the innermost layer. The outer sheaths create the human being—you can think of your body as the holder of consciousness.

The Body Sheath (Annamaya Kosha)

This layer is derived from food. This is our physical body, made up of what we eat. If we do not eat to keep our doshas in check, it will appear on this kosha as skin disorders, disease, sallowness, and weakness. In the physical body, it's easy to be confused and assume that we are separate from each other. The illusion that we are all separate gives rise to suffering and isolation. As we go deeper into the layers, we see how this can be our protective covering, but we must also remain open to new ideas, new foods, new activities, and new ways of thinking.

The Energy Sheath (Pranamaya Kosha)

This layer is derived from prana, our life force. Under the Annamaya kosha lies this kosha, which supports the bodily functions. The breath, or prana, unites us with all sentient beings, including people, animals, flowers, and trees—all creation. When we connect to our prana, we can drop the illusion of isolation and feel the connectedness to all things. Prana keeps us alive, so we must nurture it and be aware of caring for it. Breath work brings us into the practice of nurturing and cultivating prana.

The Mind Sheath (Manomaya Kosha)

This is the mental body. Comprising the mind, this kosha resides in the most constricted part of the body—we literally think too much, allow ourselves to rely on those thoughts or thoughts from others to define our goals, aspirations, and beliefs, and this can restrict us from our soul-centered choices for ourselves.

This sheath tricks us into believing our senses and emotions, and if we are really constricted, we believe what others think of us and allow that to rule our lives. To reach the level of pure conscious awareness, we need to break free of this barrier and allow ourselves to look deeply within, drop the narrative of our lives, and get to know and trust our true essence of being. You are limited only by your imagination in this kosha—so break free!

The Sheath of Intellect, Discernment, Wisdom (Vijnanamaya Kosha)

Oh, that ego—it tricks us into thinking we are other than what we truly want to be. It gets in our way when we want to move in another direction, literally talking us out of being our true selves. This is our sense of identity. We must meditate on this level to unveil who we truly are. This level is also called the I-former, creating who you are (or who you believe you are). By discerning the information we receive, we can decide what is right for us—not just because someone told us so, but because we truly believe it for ourselves.

The Bliss Sheath, the True Self (Anandamaya Kosha)

Ah, *ananda* means "bliss" in Sanskrit. This sheath is what lies in the center of all the other layers. You can think of this as your heart center, the center of pure consciousness. This is where our true self exists, our authentic self. When we reside in this kosha, we no longer feel separation or isolation. We see the beauty of all things and find joy in every moment. The mind, intellect, and ego koshas will nudge their ways in and tell you this state of being can't possibly be true, but with meditation, yoga, and Ayurveda, you can spend more and more time here, shooing away the naysaying koshas and living in a state of pure bliss.

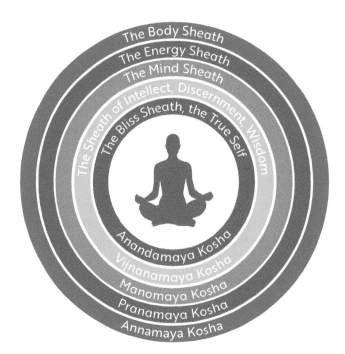

RESOURCES

24 Mantra Organic

(24mantra.com)

This Indian-based company is so far ahead of the game. Over 200 products—herbs, beans, spices, and so on—are all organic. They are also educating farmers in India (as do Banyan and Organic India) on the benefits of organic farming. I love their products, and I'm so lucky that my local Indian grocer sells them. You can also purchase online.

Amadea Morningstar

(AmadeaMorningstar.net)

Amadea is my first Ayurvedic cooking teacher and now a dear friend and co-facilitator. Her first two cookbooks, *The Ayurvedic Cookbook* and *Ayurvedic Cooking for Westerners* are a must for the Ayurvedic kitchen. Her deep knowledge and wisdom is legendary.

Ayurvedic Institute

(Ayurveda.com)

For classes and workshops in both India and the United States. Also you will find great products in their online shop. Their Super Nasya Oil and Deep Love drops are my favorites. Sign up for their newsletter.

Banyan Botanicals

(BanyanBotanicals.com)

Nearly all the herbs mentioned in the book are available from Banyan Botanicals. Their products are all organic—certified in the United States and India. There is lots of useful information on how to use the products and contraindications. In addition, their video series demonstrating various Ayurvedic practices is fantastic.

Chandi, LLC

(Chandika.com)

Home to a full spectrum of Ayurveda products formulated by Vaidya Ramakant Mishra, an Ayurvedic physician, researcher, and educator who comes from a long line of Ayurvedic experts. Most herbs are sourced in India, though some are sourced in Europe or the United States.

The Chopra Center

(Chopra.com)

This website has information on classes, workshops, online resources, and a great newsletter. My Ayurvedic journey began here.

Davidji Meditation

(Davidji.com)

Davidji uncovers the mysteries of meditation in workshops around the world. A natural teacher, his humor and delivery of information make meditation accessible to all.

Dr. John Douillard

(LifeSpa.com)

Dr. John's newsletter and videos help make complicated issues in Ayurveda easy to understand. He has incredible energy that will spur you on. Check out his books, among them *Ayurveda for Kids* and *Body, Mind, Sport*.

Floracopeia

(Floracopeia.com)

This is one of the best places for purchasing Ayurvedic essential oils.

Harish Johari

(HarishJohari.org)

Harish Johari is full of ancient Ayurvedic wisdom that's esoteric and fascinating. His book *Ayurvedic Healing Cuisine* contains wonderful recipes and Ayurvedic advice not often taught in the United States.

Maharishi Ayurveda (MAPI)

(www.mapi.com)

Vpk® by Maharishi Ayurveda provides Ayurvedic products sourced from sustainable, authentic, whole plant ingredients. Its formulations are designed to restore and maintain balance where imbalance exists.

National Ayurvedic Medical Association

(NAMA) (AyurvedaNama.org)

NAMA is working to create certification for Ayurvedic practitioners on many levels. They also have a yearly conference where you can meet some of the top Ayurvedic leaders in the world, as well as network with other practitioners. On their website. you will find resources and many video lectures on Ayurvedic topics.

Organic India

(OrganicIndiaUSA.com)

Famous for their line of Tulsi teas, Organic India also sells organic supplements and foods.

Pure Indian Foods

(PureIndianFoods.com)

My friend Sandeep Aggarwal comes from a long line of Indian ghee producers, and he makes some of the best ghee I've ever had (outside of my own!) right here in the United States. His products are all organic and top of the line, including digestive ghees (made with herbs and spices), spices, jaggery, chyawanprash, Indian spice trays, and more.

The Spice Sage

(MySpiceSage.com)

You can find hard-to-locate spices here, but they are not all organic.

REFERENCES

Abbas, Abul K., Andrew H. Lichtman, and Shiv Pillai. *Basic Immunology: Functions and Disorders of the Immune System*. 4th ed. Philadelphia: Saunders, 2012.

Aggarwal, Bharat B. *Healing Spices: How to Use 50 Everyday and Exotic Spices to Boost Health and Beat Disease*. New York: Sterling Publishing, 2011.

Ahuja, Aashna. "15 Jaggery Benefits: Ever Wondered Why Our Elders End a Meal with Gur?". NDTV. Accessed October 19, 2017. http://food.ndtv.com/health/15-jaggery -benefits-ever-wondered-why-our-elders -end-a-meal-with-gur-1270883.

American Autoimmune Related Diseases Association. "Autoimmune Disease Statistics." Accessed June 15, 2014. https://www.aarda.org /news-information/statistics.

Ayurveda For You. "These 13 Natural Urges Should Not Be Suppressed." Accessed October 19, 2017. https://www.ayurveda -foryou.com/clinical_ayurveda/urges1.html.

Bachman, Nicolai. *The Language of Ayurveda: A Reference Book of Chants, Verses, and Vocabulary*. Bloomington: Trafford Publishing, 2010.

Chakras.info. "The 7 Chakras." Accessed October 19, 2017. http://www.chakras.info /7-chakras.

The Chopra Center. "Yoga for Your Dosha." Accessed August 1, 2017. http://www.chopra .com/articles/designing-a-yoga-routine-for-your -dosha#sm.0001kfy14k7x7fbtspo1xi3eua7wr.

Chopra, Deepak. "Many Worlds and the Five Koshas." *Huffington Post*. Accessed October 19, 2017. https://www.huffingtonpost.com /deepak-chopra/many-worlds-and -the-five-_b_7475.html.

Douillard, John. "An Ayurvedic Perspective on Mood and Memory." *LifeSpa*. Accessed October 19, 2017. https://www.lifespa.com /ayurvedic-perspective-on-mood-and-memory/.

Draxe.com. Accessed October 19, 2017. http://www.draxe.com.

Earthing.com. "What Is Earthing?" Accessed October 19, 2017. https://www.earthing.com /what-is-earthing.

Frawley, David, and Sandra Summerfield Kozak, M.S. *Yoga for Your Type: An Ayurvedic Approach to Your Asana Practice*. Detroit: Lotus Press, 2001.

Group, Edward. Global Healing Center. "The Health Benefits of Sungazing." Accessed October 19, 2017. https://www.globalhealingcenter.com/natural-health/health-benefits-of-sungazing.

Insight Awareness. "Kansi Vatki Foot Massage." Accessed October 19, 2017. http://www.insightawareness.com/services/kansa-vatki.

Lad, Usha, and Dr. Vasant Lad. *Ayurvedic Cooking for Self-Healing*. Albuquerque: The Ayurvedic Press, 1994.

Lad, Vasant. *Textbook of Ayurveda: Fundamental Principles*. Albuquerque: The Ayurvedic Press, 2002.

LifeSpa. "Diet and Seasonal Eating: Seasonal Guides by Month." Accessed October 19, 2017. https://lifespa.com/category/diet-seasonal-eating.

Morningstar, Amadea, and Urmila Desai. *The Ayurvedic Cookbook*. Detroit: Lotus Press, 1990.

Pole, Sebastian. *Ayurvedic Medicine*. London: Singing Dragon Publishers, 2006.

Rosen, Richard. "10 Steps for Perfect Sun Salutations." *Yoga Journal*. Accessed October 20, 2017. https://www.yogajournal.com/poses/ray-of-light.

Singleton, Mark. "The Ancient & Modern Roots of Yoga." *Yoga Journal*. Accessed July 30, 2017. https://www.yogajournal.com/yoga-101/yoga-s-greater-truth.

Sun Gazing.com. "6 Plants That Will Make You the Healthiest and Happiest According to NASA. Accessed October 19, 2017. http://www.sun-gazing.com/6-plants-put-home-will-make-healthiest-according-nasa.

Swamij.com. "Five Sheaths or Koshas of Yoga." Accessed October 19, 2017. http://www.swamij.com/koshas.htm.

Tarkeshi, Jasmine. *Easy Poses, Guided Meditations, Perfect Peace Wherever You Are*. Emeryville, CA: Sonoma Press, 2017.

Tirtha, Swami Sadashiva. *The Ayurvedic Encyclopedia: Natural Secrets to Healing, Prevention and Longevity*. Chicago: Sat Yuga Press, 1998

Tiwari, Bri. Maya. *The Path of Practice: A Women's Book of Ayurvedic Healing, with Food, Breath and Sound*. New York: Ballantine Books, 2000.

INDEX OF PRACTICES, RECIPES, AND REMEDIES

INDEX

Brass, 109
Breath work (pranayama)
    about, 115
    Alternate Nostril Breathing (Nadi
        Shodhana), 116–117
    Bellows Breath (Bhastrika), 118
    Cooling Breath (Sheetali), 117–118
Burping, 31

C

Campaign for Safe Cosmetics, 22
Carrier oils, 91
Causal dimension, 15
Chakras
    about, 111
    crown (sahasrara), 114
    heart (anahata), 112
    root (muladhara), 111
    sacral (svadhisthana), 111–112
    solar plexus (manipura), 112
    third eye (ajna), 113
    throat (vishuddha), 113
Chanting
    about, 39
    chakra, 111–114
    cooking with mindfulness, 109
    mantra, 110
Chia seeds, 153
Chickpeas, 77–78, 154
Chyawanprash, 32, 34
Cilantro, 153
Cinnamon, 153
Circadian rhythm, 12
Cleanses, all-season, 137–139
Cloves, 153
Cooking with Mindfulness, 109
Copper, 109
Coriander, 154

Creation, 5
Cumin, 154
Curry leaves, 154

D

Daikon radish, 70, 154
Daily routines
    aromatherapy, 90–91
    drinking hot water with lemon or lime, 85
    dry brushing, 86
    head oiling, 126–127
    late fall/early winter (vata) seasonal
        adjustments, 133–134
    late winter/spring (kapha) seasonal
        adjustments, 135–136
    nasya oil, 89
    neti pot, 88
    oil massage, 86–87
    oil pulling, 84
    sample, 50–52
    summer (pitta) seasonal adjustments, 136–137
    tongue scraping, 81
    yoga, 92–105
Dhanvantari, 5
Dietary guidelines, 30–34
Digestion, 18–20, 55. *See also* Dietary guidelines
Dinacharya, 45, 50–52
Dosha. See also specific
    about, 6–7
    balancing, 38–41
    characteristics, 10–11
    doshic cycles, 12–13
    quiz, 8–10

E

Earthing, 122–123
Eating, 19. *See also* Dietary guidelines

ACKNOWLEDGMENTS

My appreciation goes out to all of the following:

My great teachers living on earth and those living on another plane who introduced me to Ayurveda and a deeper level of meditation, including Dr. David Simon, Dr. Deepak Chopra, Amadea Morningstar, Dr. John Douillard, Dr. Vasant Lad, Jennifer Ayres, Ishwari Johnson, and Dr. Ramkumar Kutty. I have been deeply influenced as well by the teachings of the Vedas, Paramahansa Yogananda, Swami Muktananda, and the teachings of Jewish meditation from Rabbi Aryeh Kaplan. You all reminded me of the knowledge I have deep inside; you helped me uncover it and share it with the world. Not only am I deeply grateful, I am also immensely happy.

My psychic friends, especially Aurora Gabriel, who told me I would be a teacher and a writer when I was just a bookstore owner.

My editor, Clara Song Lee, who asked questions, listened, and assured me along the way.

I want to thank Oprah Winfrey for hiring me as her intern at WJZ-TV in Baltimore, Maryland, when I was in high school. I like to think that she sprinkled me with fairy dust, as my life has been incredibly blessed since that time.

In addition I would like to thank my very first editor, Margery Greenfeld Morgan, at the *Jerusalem Post* in Tel Aviv, who took me under her wing and taught me so much.

All my Breathe Books and Ayurvedic clients and students who have come to me over the past 10 years for advice and support, I thank you so much for trusting me and Ayurveda to help you heal and make your life better. You have made my life better, too. I especially want to thank those who supported my endeavors over the years, including Bill Clarke, Scott Plank and Dana DiCarlo, Jannie Eisenberger, Debby Sugarman, and Ross Williams.

Our Breathe Meditation Sangha (going strong since 2009)—you are a weekly inspiration for me. I love meditating with you and probably learn far more from you than you learn from me. A deep bow of gratitude.

My mom, Bunny Singer, and my sisters, Margery Braver and Ellen Weis, who for years had no idea what to make of me and maybe still don't! Thank you for your doubts and questions, and for being great teachers to me. Love to all of you.

My mother-in-law, Mary Lou Bohlen, I thank you. Your incredibly generous support literally gave me the space to write. All my love (and thank you for your son!).

My husband, Larry Bohlen, who showed up in my bookstore one day when we were in our forties, the perfect age for soul mates to meet (in this lifetime). Our lives changed in that moment and will forever be better, stronger, and happier for it. My love for you is boundless, infinite, and joyful.

My three furry babies, Ella, Shadow, and Joonie. Ella, your Border Collie/Jack Russell wisdom teaches me to never give up and to be intense in everything, including loving and playing. Shadow, your beautiful, graceful presence teaches me to be still and in the moment. And Joonie—my rescue puppy from India—you have taught me resilience, trust, and what it means to rest in true love.

ABOUT THE AUTHOR

SUSAN WEIS-BOHLEN has a full-time practice as an Ayurvedic consultant, cooking teacher, meditation teacher, and leader of sacred site tours. She attributes her meditation, yoga, and Ayurvedic practice (and just about every good thing that has ever happened to her) to a near-death experience (NDE) at the age of 13 in 1976. After falling through a glass shower door, her left arm and leg were nearly severed, and a shard of glass caused a deep, penetrating cut to the left side of her back behind her heart. This intense experience led her to an understanding that we are much more than our bodies, and our minds can create our reality.

During the NDE, she was offered a choice—to go back or to stay where she was. After some contemplation, she chose to return to the world as she knew it. Life has been so adventurous and amazing since that day, that she is forever grateful she was given the choice to return. In fact, she sometimes wonders if she did die after all, and this incredible existence is her death experience. Hmmmm.

CPSIA information can be obtained
at www.ICGtesting.com
Printed in the USA
JSHW052151160323
38562JS00002B/2

9 781939 754172